HEAL
YOURSELF

To my dear friend Dian whose
Heart is finer than Gold —
and her mind is sparkling with
Brilliance of thoughts that
uplift others   May the Great
Spirit Guide you all the days
of your life —

Sandr

D1617107

HEAL
YOURSELF

DR. SANDOR SIGMOND

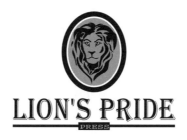

LION'S PRIDE
PRESS

BEL AIR, CALIFORNIA

Design: Suzie Dotan
Typeface - Titles: Futura Bold
Typeface - Text:: Garamond Book Condensed, Garamond Book Condensed Italic

HEAL YOURSELF

You Can!
By That
One Power
ALL LIFE
in
YOU

By Dr. Sandor Sigmond
Author of *The Book of Jade* and *Shadowscapes*

FIRST EDITION

Library of Congress Control Number: 2002111460

For information address: Lions Pride Press, P.O. Box 491956, Barrington Post Office, Los Angeles California 90049-9998

ISBN 0-9721947-0-3

i

....

THIS BOOK IS DEDICATED TO

MY DAUGHTER, SUE

AND TO THE MEMORY

OF MY SON, JEREMEY

TABLE OF CONTENTS

The

Best Teacher

The

Best Pupil

The

Best Leader

The

Best Follower

The Spirit, the Person

is something incomplete.

It imparts motion to body and mind

by refashioning the human constitution.

It belongs to the realm of quality, not quantity.

It is the inner experience which is felt

in sickness as well as in health

in sorrow as well as in joy.

It is the Current of LIFE which surges continually.

It is the Light that is found in the heart

and visibly seen in the Eye.

The Person is the Reality which is linked

to God and to each and every living being.

Asserting its presence, its freedom,

by endowing its Love to the one

who is ready to accept it!

SPECIAL THANKS

To my wife Rita—Blessed is her memory—who stood by me when things were rough, for her support over the years, when I stayed late in my office, serving the needs of my patients, and ignoring her own needs. She made many house calls with me at night - and entertained many patients in the cafeteria during our trips abroad while I worked in our room.

Special thanks to my patients who helped me to become a good doctor.

To Zev Braun who inspired me to write this book so that everyone may benefit from it.

To Beverly Werber who made many corrections and suggestions to me.

To Tracey Feirtag, whose patient and careful corrections brought the manuscript to completion.

To my editor, Michele Tempesta, whose suggestions and questions were of great benefit to me.

To Drs. Eli M. Gindi, Robert H. Landaw, T. Gregory Kirianoff, Gilbert D. Callis, and Donald Rosman, who took their time and evaluated this book frankly.

Special thanks to my daughter, Suzie Dotan, for her graphic designs and immeasurable assistance.

FOREWORD

Dr. Sandor Sigmond is a remarkable individual. My first professional encounter with Sandor was just prior to a planned operation by an orthopedist for a nerve entrapment syndrome in my forearm. He had noticed that I favored this arm, and casually asked what was wrong. He then proceeded to manipulate my forearm for one or two minutes and afforded me the first relief from discomfort in several months. After a few planned treatment visits, my pain was gone and with some special exercise instructions, I had normal use of my forearm and I cancelled my surgery.

Since then, as a practicing internist, I have sent many of my patients to Sandor with either the simplest or the most complex of musculoskeletal problems. Many return to me with stories similar to mine. Nearly all come away impressed with his unique style and approach, combining his chiropractic expertise with his personal healing style. I have seen him treat the most mundane of muscular complaints, and I have seen him help a hemiplegic man walk after being wheelchair-bound.

Sandor retired from chiropractic practice three years ago, much to the dismay of his faithful following of patients, colleagues and friends. He has spent these years writing poetry, his life story and most recently this remarkable text. His genuine and unique style is put forth in this book in much the way he might present it personally. He provides inspirational instruction in self-healing, emotional and physical balance and health maintenance. I hope you enjoy and benefit from this wonderful book written with heart and soul by a unique healer.

Elie M. Gindi, MD

PREFACE

Dr. Sandor Sigmond has been a prominent chiropractor in Los Angeles for many years. His success in treating illness and pain has brightened the lives of many grateful patients from all walks of life.

In his new book, Heal Yourself, Dr. Sigmond has succeeded in expanding his audience from those whom he has personally touched with his own hands to all people who can read and think.

Dr. Sigmond has added together his extraordinary gifts as a healer to his skills as a writer, poet, philosopher and teacher to produce a book worthy of our contemplation and study.

Using text, illustrations and self-tests, Dr. Sigmond teaches us how to heal ourselves and how to stay healthy. His teachings go beyond the physical body to the soul, and ultimately, in his words, to the "One Power—ALL LIFE— in You."

As I have highly recommended Dr. Sigmond to my patients, colleagues and friends, I now can recommend this tome to all people who care about spiritual growth and optimum health.

Robert M. Landaw, M.D.
Assistant Clinical Professor of Pediatrics
UCLA School of Medicine
July 19, 1999

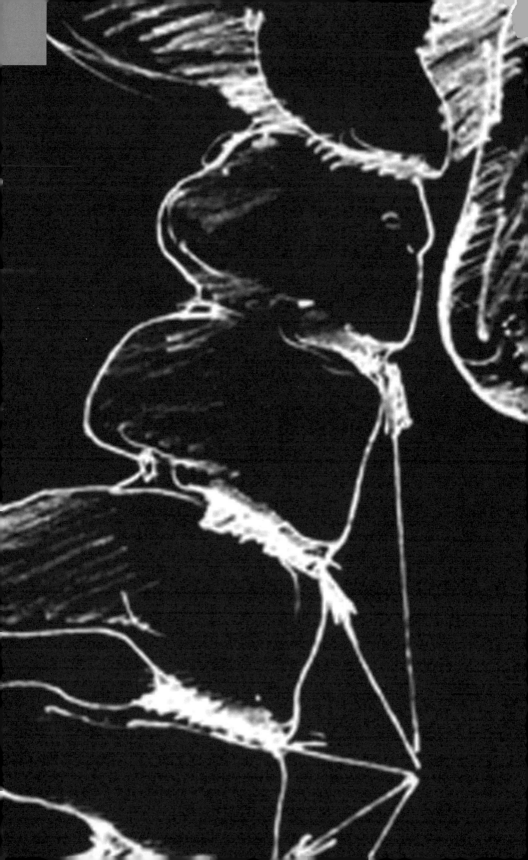

The first lesson the soul of the universe gave to all living creatures to ensure success in their journeys throughout time was MOTION. Movement is progress! All living beings must progress through movement. If you fail to make an effort, if you do not exert yourself, how do you hope to achieve your dream? How can you possibly succeed?

The soul of the universe is LIFE, which is present in everyone and in everything on earth. LIFE, being beyond description and beyond comprehension, is the potent part of each of us while the physical part of us—the body—by itself is impotent. Luckily, the two parts are one. Life needs the body as much as the body needs life, and the mind needs both. We are the mind supported by life and body.

So we must be active. Be progressive. Be constructive. Be uplifting. Be fruitful. Be grateful. Be sharing. Be considerate. Be just in our dealings. Be supportive. Be truthful. Be loving. Be peaceful.

Remember! LIFE and KNOWLEDGE is the light within all. You, as a LIFE on this earth, are a light expressing the Light of the Universe. Act accordingly and be in harmony with all living things and you will in turn be with the ALL LIFE of the Universe, the source of all.

Above all, be happy. Declare yourself to be alive, for this declaration gives you the liberty to experience yourself. Personal power is not achieved by supplication but by exerting your spirit, the same way spiritual gifts come not by exerting yourself but by waiting patiently in supplication. It is the PRESENCE OF LIFE in you that does all good things. Your mind needs to realize this for you to be successful.

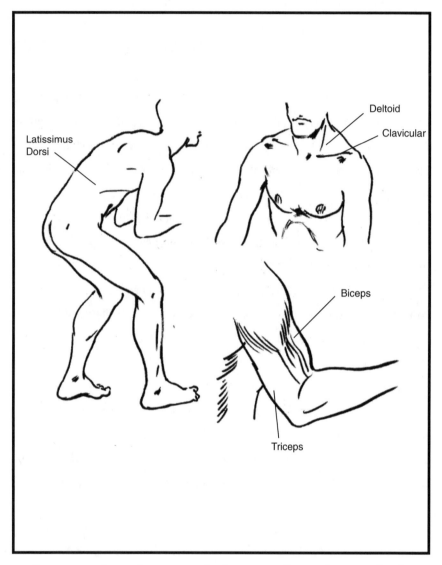

Topography of some of the muscles of your body

WHAT THIS BOOK WILL DO FOR YOU

What are the real secrets of success? Is it heredity? Is it personality? Or, is it education? Or your profession? These are all certainly important, but there is something more important than any of them. It is your ability to use your judgment consciously, to feel deeply, and to be one with that ONE LIFE that will never abandon you.

Knowing your life will help you to heal yourself.

The purpose of this book is to teach you about your body and about yourself. The book allows you to use your common sense—your deeper judgment—in evaluating your health. In this way you will be able to reconnect those areas of your being that need renewal.

The book begins with an inspirational message from three friends of the spirit of man: the honey bee, the ant, and the spider. The book is designed as a practical guide to the subject of human health, thought, and the human spirit. It avoids academic or technical jargon, yet it is based on decades of experience with my patients.

Now, let's hear the message of the three friends:

Do not harbor discontentment
Be not like a canker worm
That grows to devour.
Do not feed on your sorrows
by recounting them over and over.
For pain you cry out
And for disappointment you weep.
You feed your own shadow with shadows.
In the end you forget your connection
With Life and to Life.
With the result that you may forget that
the ALL LIFE was, is, and shall be
Your strength.

3

Learn the lessons of the honeybee, a worker in a community who stores his house with sweet provisions only. O Spirit of Man! Store your house with harmony and love.

Now listen to the ant, who is also an unselfish worker, living for the benefit of his community. He carries his burden for all and together they work to build their stores.

Let the spider teach you about the oneness of life. By the geometrical figures of unseen worlds he builds his house, needing no lessons from other spiders. He moves by the spirit within and moves in concert with the spirit of things without. The spider speaks to the spirit of man. There are two ways to knowledge before you: One is by the soul of things and the other by reason. Which one will you choose?

CHAPTER 1:

SO!

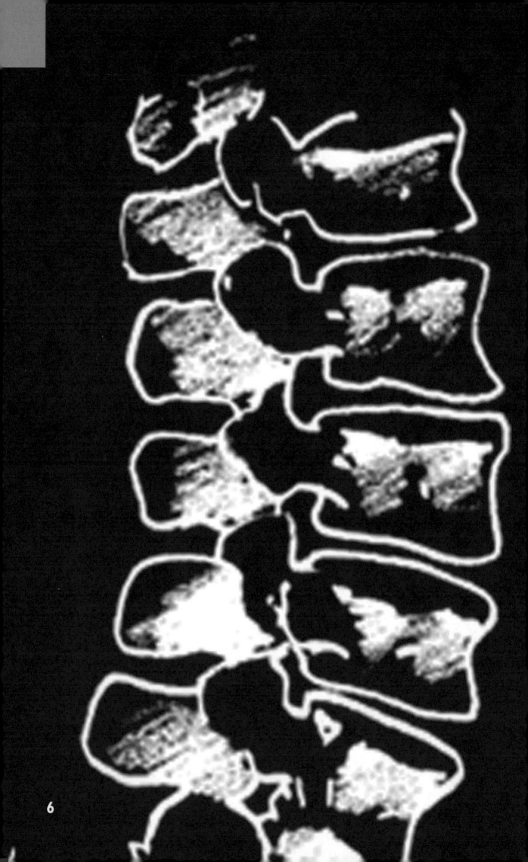

6

S o you want to heal yourself? Good. I have many times during my life. I became 82 years young on July 4, 2002. All episodes, all events in my life have made me conscious of this fact: Without the spark of spirit there can be no conscious life for me, or for anyone. That wonderful spark caused my body to heal after by-pass surgery in June 1998.

This healing was made possible by the presence of the spirit which directed my mind, its instrument to heal, and caused my body to perform incredible acts of recovery which my mind alone could not achieve. When a human being realizes that he can be alive one moment, dead the next, he wonders if there is a part of himself that is indestructible, that death cannot touch. The years have taught me that all the living are a part of the whole spectrum of life. None can exist independently or separately from the whole.

The invisible spark of the spirit that shines through the eyes of a child or adult in a moment of joy or expresses its presence in tears of sorrow or gladness is the real person in everyone.

The ever-changing physical self, with all its limitations, can be likened to an outward picture of the inner spirit, the spark that is the external part of everyone. I feel now more than ever that to live day-by-day for the elevation of the inner self, our true self, constitutes wisdom. Having reached my present age does not mean that I have stopped growing. No! It means that my physical age does not limit my spirit's power nor its aspirations nor its external possibilities. Wisdom I must earn by constant aspiration, by work and by reaching out to others and by doing good. My physical age, nor your physical age, is not and should not be a barrier to the inner spirit's life!

Did I feel alone during the experience of surgery? No! No human being is ever alone. The spark of life is with us all. One thing I learned when I was young: God is with me and His presence hovers over me and all the living. The psalmist declares (Ps. 27) "The Lord is the strength of my life; of whom shall I be afraid?" Life never neglects any one. The mind does. The mind easily loses its balance and gets confused. But one's life, never! Not even the instability of the mind affects it. Your life is a companion and faithful friend to the consciousness and its counselor.

When I felt pain in my chest or leg after open heart surgery, or when I could not take a breath, I accepted that pain by making it a part of me. Although the mind rejects its pain, I was determined to accept it. Pain is a friend. During the episodes of pain, I learned to become more appreciative of what I had in my life. I accepted the lessons of humility. My reward? I healed faster than my physicians expected.

This experience added to my understanding that was, by now, constitutional. It made clear that I had been given additional time to make good promises, which I had consciously or unconsciously neglected. This opportunity allowed me to assemble my life's experiences in this book, to leave the lessons of my experiences behind for the benefit of everyone. The giver of life is far more gracious than I deserve.

This book must shed a light of hope. You, my reader, might learn from my experiences and those of my patients.

You must progress until the last seconds at life's end.

Prior to my 78th birthday, on March 26, 1998, the anniversary of my wife's death, and against the advice and pleadings of my daughter, Sue, I entered Cedars Sinai Hospital in Los Angeles for an angiogram with the possibility of an angioplasty. When I recovered from that procedure, the cardiologists, two of them, informed me that I had a blockage at the bifurcation of the left descending artery and circumflex artery. They suggested a stent be placed in the artery or I would have to undergo a bypass.

I wanted the open heart surgery in lieu of the stent, but I allowed the cardiologists at Cedars to talk me into a new type of stent whose rate of success was but 70 percent. That's a 30 percent failure rate.

One minute the roses are blooming, giving off their sweet scent. Their beauty fills the eye of those who behold them. The next, the petals are falling. The scent is fading and the rose that was is no more. When Rita died, the world seemed dark. As her soul left, the light that was is no more.

Healing. Have I healed myself from all my experiences? The answer is yes and no. Healing is a lifetime process in which forgiveness plays an important role. And having faith in life and the Giver of life supported me, day-by-day.

Life is not static, not a measurable quantity of something. It is an influx constantly filling a void left after each event and each experience. As the psalmist said, "Have mercy upon me, O Lord, for I am weak. Oh Lord, heal me." (Psalm 6, 3) Also from Psalm 16, 5-9, "The Lord is the portion of mine inheritance and of my cup. Thou hath maintained my lot. The lines have fallen unto me in pleasant places; yea, I have a goodly heritage. I will bless the Lord who hath given me counsel; my reins also instruct me in the night seasons. I have set the Lord always before me because he is at my right hand. I shall not be moved. Therefore my heart is glad and my glory rejoyceth. My flesh also shall rest in hope."

The stent procedure was unsuccessful. After much pain and discomfort as well as worry for me and my family, I had open heart surgery. As a result of the open heart surgery, my body has been subjected to severe trauma. During the healing process, which took about five weeks, I experienced a variety of post-operative discomforts. After four days at home I had to return to Cedars to remove fluid from around my heart. I stayed over night. When I entered the hospital the second time I weighed 182 pounds. After they removed the fluid I lost 10 pounds. This is a normal reaction to open heart surgery. Some patients may experience constipation. I did not. I did have pain during movements or when I coughed. I held a small pillow to my chest to relieve my chest wall discomfort.

My right leg was swollen at the ankle where a vein was removed. I experienced fatigue in the first two weeks of recovery. It soon disappeared when I increased my walking regimen. I did not experience forgetfulness, a normal response after such trauma.

My emotional response to the entire process was as important to me as the surgery itself.

I had witnessed my wife's episode in 1992, and so was aware that the same helplessness could lead to depression. I did not allow myself to sink into that. The fatigue

I experienced put temporary limitations on me, and I was not concerned with my sexuality or having to go back to work. These can be a great concern after returning from the hospital.

The greatest weapons I used against depression was writing and being active both physically and mentally. For the first month I had a helper stay with me in my home. I felt an increase in my heartbeat whenever I was on my left side or when I was lying flat. So, I slept sitting up. This way I avoided the throbbing sensation in my ears. I elevated my leg higher than the level of my heart to avoid swelling in my right leg. I avoided crossing my legs at the knees or ankles so not to interfere with circulation. I called my physician when I had shortness of breath. So should you. I called him when I experienced palpitations, racing heart beats. I watched my weight for a sudden increase or persistent discomfort. I was given steroids for this.

I had to modify my eating habits and now follow a low-sodium diet, and eat foods low in cholesterol to minimize future heart problems. Cholesterol can narrow the arteries through plaque formation and cause a heart attack. Cholesterol is a waxy fat-like substance that builds up in the arteries and contributes to atherosclerosis. It is found in animal products, liver, egg yolks and shrimp. I maintain the body weight appropriate for my age and height.

I recommend you keep the saltshaker out of the kitchen. If you retain water, added salt will make it difficult for your heart to force the increased volume of water through your body.

TO AVOID CONSTIPATION:

1. Increase your activity slowly
2. Avoid too much pain medication
3. Be careful of the constant use of laxatives. These decrease the natural mobility of your bowel
4. Avoid emotional stress, not just during your recovery but at all times
5. Make good use of the time given you; enjoy life to its fullest

6. Eat fresh fruits daily

7. Eat leafy vegetables

8. Drink six to eight glasses of fluid a day

Become more physically active during and after you recover. This will help to improve your heart's efficiency, its muscle tone, its strength and, above all, your outlook on life. When you are physically active, you have hope and a sense of self-reliance.

When I was young I had to walk long distances. I was born in a rural township of 4,000 families and everyone walked as their mode of transportation. I taught all of my patients to walk—not by miles but by time. Time equals miles. Walk minutes, the distance will take care of itself. Increase the minutes and you will be surprised how much distance you have covered.

Walk with joy in your step. Do not walk with tolerance. Do it because walking will insure that you live! And you will live a good life. Walk on a flat area. Do not wear yourself out. I live in a hilly area so I had someone drive me to a mall where I could walk. Do not walk immediately after eating. Pace yourself. Your body will warn you when to stop your activity and rest.

When you experience palpitations or shortness of breath, or when you feel dizzy or weaker than usual, call your physician!

Exercise is the sum total of daily activity that includes mental, physical and emotional activity. Perform these exercises slowly at least two times a day. Do not exercise for an hour after eating.

SITTING:

1. Straighten each knee, lifting from floor. Then lower it.

2. Lift each knee toward your chest, then lower it.

3. Bend your arms at the elbows and straighten.

   Do not do any exercises with your neck to avoid dizziness.

· ·

4. Lift your hands overhead, then lower.

STANDING:

1. Place hands on hips. Twist right, then left.
2. Extend arms at your side. Bend to the right and then to the left.
3. Bend and straighten knees with feet on the floor.
4. Walk in place.

EXERCISE UP TO FIFTEEN MINUTES DAILY.

Are you vulnerable to coronary heart disease?

Look for these signs:

1. ***Heredity.*** If your family has a history of coronary artery disease, it predisposes you to develop the disease.
2. ***Smoking.*** Smoking makes your heart beat faster, raises blood pressure and narrows the arteries, increases the workload of your heart, and prevents red blood cells from carrying oxygen to the heart muscle.
3. ***Overweight.*** This predisposes you to develop high blood pressure, diabetes and elevated cholesterol.
4. ***Cholesterol.*** This is manufactured by your body and is also found in various foods. When you take in more than your body needs, the excess may be deposited in your arteries and cause atherosclerosis.
5. ***Emotional Stress.*** Continued stress increases your heart rate, your blood pressure, irregularities of your heartbeat, your blood pressure and cholesterol.
6. ***High Blood Pressure.*** High blood pressure has two effects: the growth of fatty deposits in the coronary arteries and the increase in the workload of the heart as it pumps.
7. ***Lack of Exercise.*** Remember exercise by itself will not prevent or cure heart disease, but if you are living a sedentary lifestyle, you may increase the risk of a

heart attack. If you exercise it will reduce the risk as well as modify your high blood pressure.

8. **Diabetes.** You need to control the level of your blood sugar.

REDUCE HARMFUL STRESS: A MUST

Stress is a fact of life. In one sense stress prepares you for unfamiliar and threatening situations. This is your body's reaction to physical, emotional and environmental circumstances that frighten, excite, confuse or just irritate you. However, too much stress can have an adverse effect.

This is what you need to do:

1. Change your habits and mode of living.
2. Relax your body and mind daily.
3. Read a book. Use music to relax.
4. Take a midday rest at work or at home.
5. Exercise regularly.
6. Walk and walk away from stressful situations.
7. Reduce stress in your life.
8. Pray. May the meditation of your heart be acceptable, even by yourself from yourself. All healing depends on how close you are to your true self. Do not erect obstacles between yourself and your essential self.

SEX: IS IT ON YOUR MIND?

The desire for the resumption of sexual intimacy begins within 21 to 28 days after surgery. In my case I had to wait much longer, which was good. For such activity should be resumed gradually.

When you are able to work around the house without discomfort or walk three to four miles, sexual activity may be contemplated. Before then, you can touch your love and caress each other. All these are part of sexual activity and should be a source of comfort and hope for the renewal of life.

When you do resume sexual intimacy, choose the position of comfort. All other activities in bed could cause irregular heart rhythms. Before you resume sexual intimacy, discuss it with your cardiologist or your internist, especially if you were given medication for an arrhythmia.

Be careful not to take unsafe heart stimulants such as mood-altering drugs. These increase your heart rate as oxygen makes more demands on your heart muscle.

If you are a woman and want to have children, speak to your physician and cardiac surgeon. Discuss with your doctor when it is safe to try to become pregnant.

DO YOU KNOW YOUR HEART?

You should understand your heart so that you will take care of it by changing your lifestyle.

Your heart is an organ composed of muscle. It is the size of your closed fist and weighs about a half-pound. It is contained in a sac known as the pericardium and contains a small amount of fluid. This fluid lubricates your heart during its movement. The muscle of your heart is called myocardium.

Your heart is divided into four chambers. A muscular wall called the septum divides your heart into a right and left side. The two upper chambers consist of a right and left atrium (collecting chambers). The two lower chambers consist of a right and left ventricle (pumping chambers).

The movement of your blood through the atrial chambers to the ventricular chambers is governed by two valves: the tricuspid valve and the mitral valve. When the ventricle chambers contract, the tricuspid and mitral valves close and prevent blood from returning to the atrium.

The flow of your blood to your lungs and your body is directed by two valves, the pulmonic valve and the aortic valve. During the time your ventricle chambers are contracting, the pulmonic and aortic valves are opened. After contraction, these valves close to prevent blood from flowing back to the pulmonary artery and aorta.

The oxygen and nutrients that your heart muscle needs come from the blood that circulates through a network of coronary arteries. They originate from a trunk of your aorta and travel on the surface of your heart before it branches into the heart muscle itself.

A reminder: You have been through a very stressful experience. The worst is over. Now begin to move on so you can return to normal life. Get rid of your stress!

Here is a word of advice to your spouse, relative or friend:

1. Don't be over protective.
2. Help in overcoming stress.
3. Have a sympathetic ear. That is, listen! not just hear sounds coming your way.
4. If the patient/loved one is angry, hostile, or depressed, encourage him or her to face up to those feelings.
5. Stress affects people of all ages and all levels of society. Stress takes may different forms. It usually comes about by an unwanted, undesired change that must be accepted involuntarily. Stress is emotional, mental and physical, such as a relationship or an event of some kind that brings on the manifestation of anger, anxiety and excitement. Yet, not all stress is bad. Happiness is a form of stress, such as the celebration of a wedding or the birth of a child. You must learn to cope with stress.
6. Too much stress makes it difficult to adopt a healthy lifestyle.
7. Under stress, the blood pressure rises, the adrenaline flows, breathing increases and the heart rate speeds up. The muscles become tense and can cause a headache, neck ache and back ache.
8. Anxiety leads to feelings of helplessness that lead to anger and irritability.
9. Stress affects everyone! Even you.

Before you begin each chapter, try to answer the quiz questions that precede it. This way, you will pre-test your knowledge about your body, and discover how much—or how little—you know about yourself. After you have read a chapter, don't read further until you have retaken the quiz. Compare your early answers with your new insights. I'm sure you will be pleased with what you learned.

Don't rush; take your time. The words will not disappear. They will wait for you! Remember, patience will lead you to understand, and understanding will lead you to knowing. Knowing becomes the foundation to right living, right thinking, right feeling, and, lastly, to right being! And, being a person is the greatest success of all!

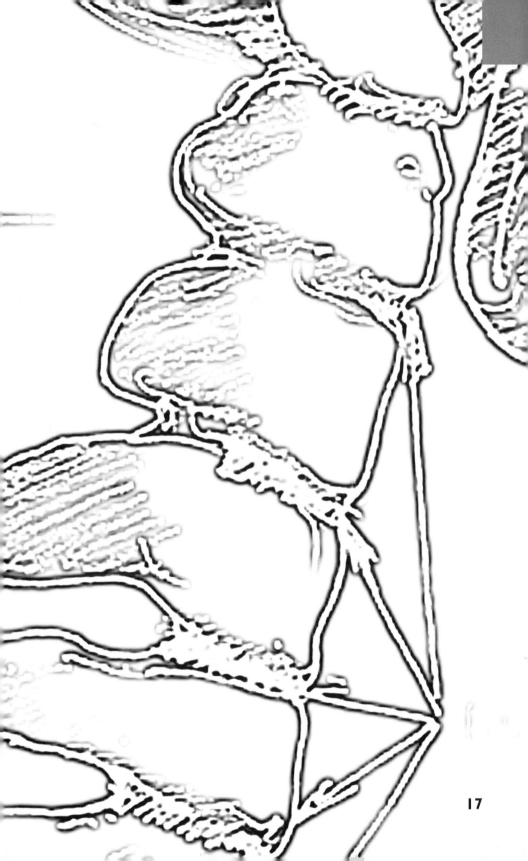

17

CHAPTER 2: NOW TEST YOURSELF

Please use a separate sheet of paper.

1. What is a joint lesion or subluxation?

2. Why do you need a case history?

3. What is spirit?

4. How is inner peace acquired?

5. How do you acquire happiness?

6. How do you keep your body in balance?

7. Why is exercise important?

8. What are you to do with your enemy?

9. What is progress?

CHAPTER 2:

BODY BALANCE

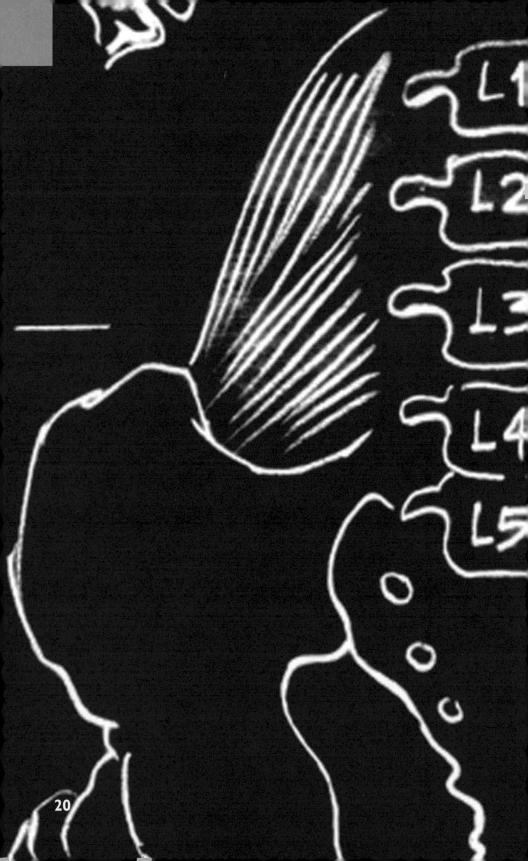

L1

L2

L3

L4

L5

A s a chiropractic doctor my concern was the preservation and restoration of health of my patients. Now that I am retired, I am concerned with educating you about how to preserve and restore your health the chiropractic way.

I have primarily focused my attention on joint lesions, or subluxations, especially in the spine. A lesion or subluxation is complex, composed of structural, functional, and/or pathologic joint changes, which will affect the integrity of the nerves and blood vessels that influence internal organs and their functions.

Your case history will help your doctor determine the care you need. Of course, you should know the reason why you are seeking chiropractic care, indeed, any medical care. You should be aware of when your symptoms began to manifest. You should always have with you the history of your health and your family history, as well as your occupational history, in case of emergency. This information will help your physician determine your safe and proper care.

Remember, you are the important person; the doctor is there to serve you.

What should be included in your history? Your age and gender, occupation, primary reason you seek care, secondary reason, chief complaint, effects of trauma, and if there is a sleeping position that helps you.

When you go to a chiropractor, you will note that he/she uses his hands to examine you. Hands are the tools of the chiropractor. He will palpate, that is, feel through the hand, as he tries to help you. He will locate areas of abnormal movement in a segment or segments within your spine.

All doctors are trained to render proper care to their patients. Anything you do with your hand is considered chiropractic, but remember that you are not trained as a chiropractic doctor.

In this book, you will be given instructions on how to help yourself at home or when you travel. These instructions will help you to maintain your health or regain and then maintain your health.

You are alive, and you are filled with energy. Your power lies in your movements of the body and within the body, mind, and your emotions. As the universe expresses its power and wisdom in the motion which is within it and around it, so do you express your power and wisdom in movement in your daily life. How you use your power is up to you alone. That is, how you care for yourself, or how you neglect yourself, is up to you.

It is important for you to take care of your body, your mind, your emotions, and your spirit. My definition of the spirit is everything that is capable of love, being just, sharing, being good, considerate, able to express loving kindness, being truthful, uplifting, and caring for others and caring for oneself without hurting others. This knowledge urges you to venerate your being, which includes taking care of your body the same way you take care of your mind or emotions. If you neglect to take care of any one of these, you splinter your power and affect your judgment at the same time.

You must remain in harmony within yourself and your surroundings. You must aspire to the highest and best in everything in your daily activities. Honor yourself each day, each moment.

Inner peace must be learned. Follow the deep relaxation exercise that begins by mentally traveling through your own body.

First, lie down and loosen all your clothing. Take a couple of slow deep breaths and relax. Let your body melt into your bed or sofa. Next, take a deep breath and hold it. Tense your entire body. Hold it for as long as you can. Then exhale and let all the tension leave you. Repeat, but this time let the tension be only half as tight. Do this exercise four times but without tensing your body. Feel the rhythm of your heart; slow it down to a regular beat. Now imagine yourself outside your body, looking in, and becoming smaller and smaller until you feel able to enter through your forehead and relax your mind. Then flow down your neck from there to one shoulder and then the other shoulder, and relax. Your body should feel warmth from the love you are giving it. If you are concerned with any part of your body, go there and give it your love.

When you have finished taking care that all your body is loved, resume your normal size inside your body. Then resume your normal self-awareness but now feeling more relaxed and confident.

Trust your life. Trust yourself. Share yourself. Be ready to help someone. In giving yourself, you will grow in every way. Keeping yourself from others will lead to loneliness and ill health. Happiness comes by sharing. Do not become isolated. Reach out, and someone will take your hand into theirs. As you reach out you will be received by life—the All Life.

Keeping your body in balance is very important. Certain areas in your body may have lost balance early in life. Therefore you should become acquainted with your body, its mechanics, and the workings of your muscles. This way you will know how to avoid the many strains and pains and ordinary aches.

Rule #1: Keep your muscles in good tone at all times. This will prevent structural and organic displacements from occurring.

Rule #2: Effort produces accomplishment. This means that you should use what you have in order for you to maintain good health.

Rule #3: You will lose what you fail to use. You use certain muscles daily, regardless of your lack of effort. But the areas you do not use are the areas you must make a concerted effort to use, because what you lose through negligence is very difficult to recover!

Exercise is important to maintain proper balance. You should understand your skeleton, the ligaments, and the muscles you use during exercise. It takes months for a good athlete to train for one performance. Even a good musician trains daily so that his/her muscles move in harmony. And, of course, an army without training will lose the battle and ultimately the war. You must prepare yourself not just physiologically but mentally and emotionally for good health. Train yourself to be healthy today.

Rule #4: Your muscles will be developed properly when they can handle your body weight effectively. All exercise should make it possible for you to handle your own weight with ease.

THE FOLLOWING EXERCISES WILL DEVELOP YOUR MUSCLES TO
HANDLE YOUR BODY WEIGHT:

1. Push-ups. Try it on the doorway. (See illustration in Chapter 12.)
2. Climbing a rope.
3. Walking uphill or walking at a fast pace.
4. Chinning. Pull yourself up on the frame of a door.
5. Lifting or moving another person of equal weight a few feet.

    If you are over 55, see your doctor for a physical exam before attempting any exercise regimen. If you are over 25, chances are that your abdominal muscles are not adequately developed. Unfortunately, eating is not the best exercise for this problem!

    If you enjoy bowling or playing golf, that's good. But these activities do not provide adequate muscle development. In my practice of several decades, I advocated walking and certain additional muscle development exercise to prevent back pain (these exercises follow in a later chapter).

POINTERS FOR DEVELOPING AND RETAINING YOUR HEALTH

1. Begin each day with gratitude: Life has returned to your physical self.
2. Put a smile on your face—you may learn to like it—and begin to exercise.
3. Motivate yourself to do something good, something constructive this day. You have the power to make decisions that benefit everyone.
4. Respect yourself and appreciate your talents, the gifts life holds for you.
5. Reach out to someone. Share yourself: lend a hand to those who need you. Sow goodness of heart this day.
6. Know when to seek assistance from family, from friends, from your physician, from strangers, and even from someone you think may be your enemy. Be gracious in your acceptance.
7. Do not take your body, your mind, your strength, or your health for granted. You cannot afford to lose any one.

8. Accept the enemy inside of you—selfish desires, anger, and hate—and the one you perceive to be outside of you because you perceive yourself in others.

9. Accept your pains as your friends. You may benefit from their presence.

10. Examine your beliefs, as these can cause illness.

11. Seek to progress every moment you have! This desire is a gift to you from All Life. Remember! You are never, never alone.

Dissatisfaction maintains the constant
Movement of progress in and through life
Progress is not a fixed state

CHAPTER 3 EXAMINATION: NOW TEST YOURSELF

Please use a separate sheet of paper.

1. What must guide you in getting well?

2. What is the best defense against sickness?

3. How much stress should you put on your body?

4. What are the anatomical areas of your spine?

5. In what position is your spine in stress?

6. What keeps your spine erect?

7. What determines how a segment of vertebrae functions?

8. When are you most prone to injury?

9. Which area of your back is weakest in its articulations?

10. What are the simple movements of your neck?

11. Which vertebrae cannot move backward?

12. What kind of motion is desirable in your sacroiliac?

13. Which area of your back makes it possible for you to bend backward or forward?

14. What areas of your back may give you the greatest trouble?

CHAPTER 3:

STAY HEALTHY THE CHIROPRACTIC WAY

As

Wisdom cannot tell

What wisdom is

And

Reason what reason is

so

Man cannot tell

What man is

and

Man cannot tell

What the ALL LIFE is.

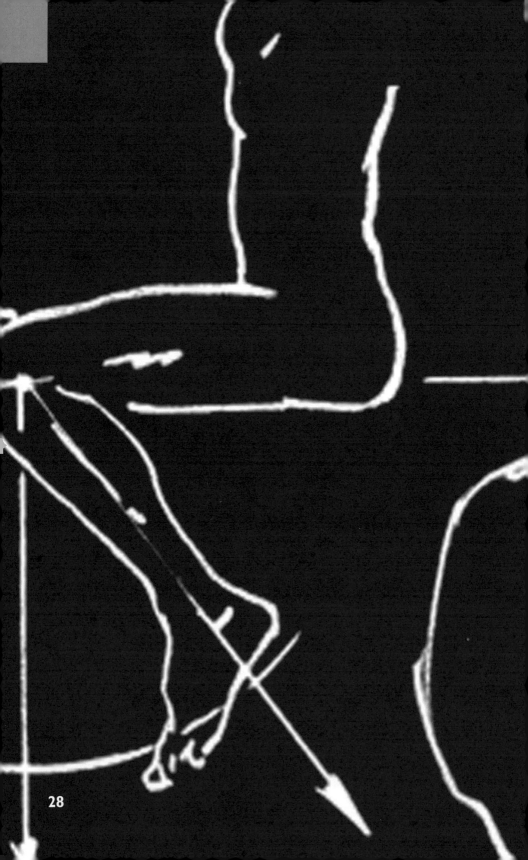

Relaxation from tension

Use this tension release exercise daily, especially after work when you are free to spend a few quiet moments on your own.

Lie down on a sofa or on your bed without a pillow under your head. You can also do this exercise seated at your desk. A pillow under your head flattens your trachea and cuts back the normal air flow to your lungs, diminishing the flow of oxygen to your brain and other vital organs.

This exercise will help you to dispense with sleeping pills or muscle relaxants.

Make sure you are comfortable.

1. Place your right or left hand (whichever is most comfortable) under your occiput (the back of your head).

2. Place the index finger of your free hand in the middle of your forehead. Press slightly downward. Imagine or visualize that your finger has pierced your skull and now is touching the palm of the hand under your head. Lie this way for about 2 minutes.

3. Now remove both hands and place them by your side. Rest for 3-5 minutes more.

4. If you do not fall asleep you will certainly be more relaxed. This is the aim: relaxation.

We are in the new millennium. Much progress has been made in the fields of medicine, in hygiene, and in the fields of chiropractic and homeopathy. The public is health-conscious and no longer willing to believe that allopathic medicine is all-knowing. Old foundations are continually being re-examined and discarded.

Not every physician knows everything about the human body or the human being. But a good physician will tell you that medicine can do only so much and you, the patient, must help yourself to prevent illness. You must protect the state of your health, and if you do become ill, you must take an active role in your recovery and treatment.

Your body's defenses must be strong enough to take over when the effects of medication cease. Your good judgment must guide you in getting well and in finding ways to maintain your good health.

Your body is an outward picture of you. You can only prove your existence through your body. If you neglect the body, you neglect yourself. You neglect the body if you allow the self to drive the body relentlessly. The body will break down sooner or later. But if you are in harmony with yourself, your body has the ability to throw off most conditions that attack it. For instance, the white blood cells have the ability to destroy viruses and bacteria. Your system produces antibodies that neutralize the invading hosts, but their success depends on a state of harmony between the self and your body. This is "health."

A heart without kindness and joy
Is weak in spirit
And without strength
There is no growth.

YOUR HEALTH DEPENDS UPON:

1. The number of white blood cells, their strength, and, in an emergency, how fast you can manufacture them in your body.

2. How quickly specific antibodies can be created against infection. The major organs involved are your liver, bone marrow and spleen.

3. The antibodies must be delivered to those areas in your body where they are needed. The delivery system is your blood, the giant river and its tributary rivulets that reach every part of your body.

4. The blood vessels must be kept in good condition. This is the job of the nervous system.

5. The state of health of the tissues being attacked and the strength of your cells and their ability to replace damaged tissues.

Health depends on each person's state of harmony. One person may become ill more often than another, and one person may recover faster than another. It is your duty to yourself to maintain good health in your blood circulation in order to prevent heart problems, strokes, and the formation of ulcers. It is also your duty to build up the strength of your bones so that they can serve you better as you age. This will help you avoid broken hips, pelvis, legs, or fractures of the vertebrae in your back and neck.

You should not stress your back by carrying more than it can handle or by running for exercise, which jars each segment and causes tears in the ligaments, not just in the back but in the knees, hips, and ankles. (More about these later.)

Life has given you the potential to maintain a healthy mind and body, but you alone must assume the responsibility for maintaining and retaining your good health, in harmony or balance within yourself. Hurt the body by abusing it through wrongful living, drugs, alcohol, exercise done incorrectly exceeding your body's abilities, or excesses of any kind, then you are abusing your very self. You choose and your life obeys and builds your body accordingly or destroys it at your command. Be mindful of what you tell yourself. Your life is your greatest of servants. Create harmony, create a state of balance between your self and your body; then your life will keep you healthy.

Increase your knowledge about your body so that you can help yourself.

Beware

As to what you accept!

I understand that what my profession has added to the overall knowledge of medicine is that there are lesions within the spine, and that their correction is necessary to restore the balance (homeostasis) in the body. These lesions and the movements of the spine are physiologic and require some anatomical knowledge. I will not deal with specifics, as this book is not intended as a textbook but a guide to health for everyone. There are too many misconceptions about the best way to keep healthy and to exercise.

The discussion about the physiological movement of your back is based on my assumption that you are somewhat familiar with basic anatomy acquired through personal experience. You may have had lumbago, sciatica, or back pain in some form. Or you may have gained this knowledge through reading; or you have known someone with back problems. You must have some basic information about the spine. It is composed of three anatomically distinct areas: the cervical (neck), thoracic (upper back), and lumbar (low back). You need to understand how these areas behave under normal conditions as you function each day.

It is impossible to fully appreciate your spine in the upright posture when you are standing, walking, dancing, or exercising without first viewing it in the horizontal position, when you are on your back or when you try to walk on your hands and feet (lizards and alligators walk in the pronograde state). If you were required to function in a horizontal position, your body's load would be carried on strong, compact, tiny bones called facets. In this condition, the intervertebral ligaments, or discs, which are flexible in nature and allow free movement of your spine, would not become torn from compression as they do not yield easily to force. Staying on your back, there would be no displacement, or subluxations in the spine. You would have a perfectly healthy back. But who could live flat on his back? Obviously, the human frame was not designed to stay horizontal forever.

Let us see what happens when you are standing erect. Here your back's mechanics are quite different. Your back is composed of bones held together by ligaments that wobble from side to side, going forward or backward. They seem to be in a state of constant instability from the beginning of life's journey to its end. In this position your spine is under constant stress. The discs between each vertebra move constantly, forever in a state of restlessness. So, don't blame yourself if you are feeling restless in life!

Clearly, your back under normal conditions is not stable. This means that there is no such thing as normal posture. Don't let anyone tell you that your posture is wrong, as everyone's back is under constant pressure.

To keep your back erect and stabilize it so that you can function, you are required to think straight. Since you have to think straight to walk straight—you do it every second of your life—why not apply the same principle in other areas of your life as well? When you think straight, you are using movement and leverage to achieve the erect posture.

Your spine moves physiologically when each vertebra moves in harmony with the one above it and the one below it; for example, the lumbar or low back moves in harmony with the sacrum and the ilia below it, and above it with your rib cage, and the rib cage with your neck. When you are experiencing limited motion in one area of your spine, the individual segment is not in harmony with its neighbor. To correct this, you must reverse the movement to correct the distortion. The same principle applies in your family and business life: Your body is your best teacher.

When we were young, we were told that man was not intended to walk upright; but our teachers didn't realize that each segment of the vertebra was shaped differently. The form of each segment determines how it will function. Each area of the spine is different and behaves differently: The lumbar vertebrae could not function well in the neck or the vertebrae in your neck could not function well in your lumbar area.

WHAT IS THE NORMAL MOVEMENT OF YOUR SPINE?

You have two main movements of your back. The first is extension, which separates two ends of an arc formed by your vertebrae. The second is the opposite: flexion. When you extend your spine, you decrease the normal existing curve in any area of your spine—remember, you have three areas: the cervical (the neck), the thoracic (upper back), and the lumbar (lower back)—while flexion will increase the normal existing curve. When you bend forward to pick up something from the floor or to tie your shoes, or when you bend backwards, when you bend sideways or when you rotate your body one way or another or each part separately—each of these positions increase or decrease the normal position of your spine. Neutral position of any area of your spine is the position between the beginning of flexion and the beginning of extension. A neutral position in life is when you make no commitment to anything; but your body, with every movement it makes, makes a commitment to perform right. Do the same in your life.

The normal curves in your back are never completely gone when you extend your back or any area in your spine. They retain some degree of anatomical flexion or forward bend.

In your lower back, in the lumbar, there is very little side-bending or rotation. You are more prone to injure yourself when you try to do things from the position of extension than when you do things from the position of flexion. To illustrate: When you extend your neck while having your hair washed at a salon, and you try to move your head suddenly, you are more likely to injure yourself than when your neck is flexed, that is, when your head is in a forward position and you wash your hair yourself.

You have vertebral arteries going up inside your cervic (neck) vertebrae to your brain. These arteries are surrounded by a group (plexus) of nerves. These enter the skull (head) through the foramen magnum (opening in back of your head) to form the basilar artery. They are prone to injury while your neck is extended. A small plaque can break off inside your blood vessels and lodge in your brain causing a stroke. Never allow yourself to be manipulated or massaged on your neck while it is extended (backward bent position). Ladies! You have been warned.

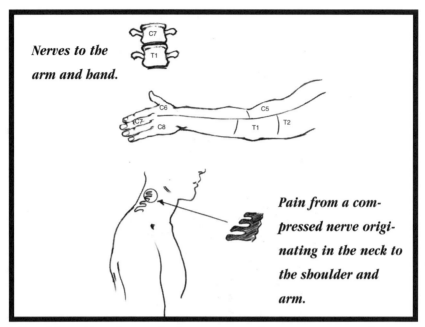

Nerves to the arm and hand.

Pain from a compressed nerve originating in the neck to the shoulder and arm.

The distribution of the nerves from your neck (cervical spine) to your hand

YOUR RIB CAGE

The upper back or thoracic cage was never meant to be as flexible as the lumbar or cervical areas. Your upper back in its articulations is the weakest area of your spine. For this reason, they are well supported by the ribs. When any amount of rotation occurs, this results in joint strain and the distortion of the vertebrae and the discs. These predispose this area to scoliosis.

Your upper back is able to make two kinds of simple movements, extension and flexion, and two kinds of combination movements, extension-rotation-sidebending and flexion-sidebending-rotation.

As your upper back is not as flexible, at the same time it is the weakest area, so when you pull out your chest to exert yourself as an individual having certain rights, remember the next person can pull out and exert his chest to exert his right as well. But as you have witnesses, so has he. Be therefore considerate of each other.

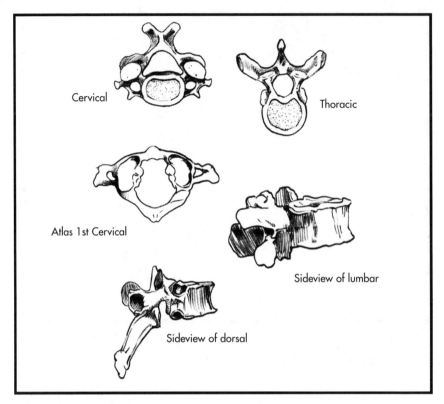

Cervical

Thoracic

Atlas 1st Cervical

Sideview of lumbar

Sideview of dorsal

The shape of the various vertebrae

YOUR CERVICAL SPINE

The bones in your neck have two divisions: from the second and including the seventh vertebrae, and the axis, atlas, and occiput. Your cervical vertebrae are perfectly adapted to the horizontal posture and you can elevate your head and bend this area up to 45 degrees. Beyond this angle, injury begins.

The upper part of your neck from the second-third and the third-fourth vertebrae operate in a forward-backward angle of about 45 degrees. From the third-fourth downward, the plane of operation becomes more perpendicular. As a result of this mechanical difference, you have the ability to rotate your neck.

Your neck has two simple movements which are bending backward, called extension, and forward-bending, called flexion. Your neck also has two compound movements: backward movement-sidebending-rotation and forward bending-rotation-sidebending.

As the smallest bones of your spine support your head, so let the gentlest part of yourself support your judgment.

THE ATLAS

This structure permits your head excessive rotation: some forward bending and backward bending and very slight side bending. This atlas is the first vertebra upon which your skull rests. It is on the basis of the structure of this joint that contortionists are able to rotate their heads in such extraordinary manner. The atlas is the only vertebra that can move forward on its base, and it is the only one that cannot move backward. This is because the second vertebra imposes on it in a projectile called the odantoid process.

In mythology it was said that the bull that supports the world will be slaughtered when the world will be at peace. The two horns of the bull that support the world will not be called the atlas of the world but will be called the horns of light. Therefore, the light of good judgment supports all of your undertakings daily.

THE MOVEMENTS OF YOUR SACRUM-OH THAT SACROILIAC PAIN!

Your sacrum is part of your pelvis structurally, but physiologically it is part of your lumbar spine. The motions of your sacrum are similar to the other segments of lum bar vertebrae. Contrary to other joints in the body, the limited motion in your sacroiliac is desirable because it increases the stability of your spine.

Please consider your infants if they fall. Check their pelvis, especially, when you see that they have a toe-in appearance with both of their feet, as the base of their sacrum is affected and the infant may compensate this way.

....

SUMMARY OF THE PHYSIOLOGIC MOVEMENT OF YOUR SPINE

The normal curves in your neck and lower back must be operative. These are known as lordatic.

The neutral position of your spine is where the facets of the vertebrae touch each other and begin to engage each other prior to either bending forward and backward.

Flexion, or forward bending, is the increase of the normal existing curve of many areas of your spine.

Extension, or backward bending, is the decrease of an existing curve of any area of your spine.

SPINAL LESION

Spinal lesion is any position and/or condition of your spinal joints that interferes with perfect function of your spine in a localized area or remotely in other areas of your body, or predisposes to types of interference. You may have been told that faulty posture or physical or mental fatigue, violence, or physical irritation can cause a lesion. But a lesion is usually the result of an exaggeration of a physiological movement in which the joint surfaces pass beyond their normal range and may become locked. In other words, a lesion occurs when you bend beyond your back's ability to bend or when you lift beyond the power of your spine's ability, when you push beyond your ability, when you become careless with yourself.

The principal factors that control the mechanical behavior of your spine are:
1. Gravity load
2. The condition of the facets in your spine
3. The shape of the bodies of the vertebrae
4. The muscular and ligamentar tensions

For example, let us say that you moderately extended your lumbar and rotated it. (In a neutral state, the structure of your lumbar will permit about 10 degrees side bend.) Let us say that your sidebending is severe. Now it has caused a strain. The dominant movement is a sidebending joint strain. And when you twist or rotate, your dominant movement is rotation or twisting or rotation sidebending.

Your ability to treat a lesion successfully is your own ability to determine the cause of your problem and diagnose it properly before you seek help from a professional. You must realize that each vertebra performs according to the structure and condition of its particular articulation and, under normal conditions, travels over a well-defined path or track. Your spine takes a terrific amount of abuse and often gets into trouble either from wear and tear or sudden strain. Our physiologic movements become jammed and then our spine has casualties in various segments all along its length.

The greatest amount of trouble in your back is between the 11th and 12th thoracic and the lumbar #1 articulations. This is the area that makes it possible for you to bend forward and backward. If you should rotate at this level of your back, you will experience a strain. This area can rotate very little, and, if you side bend, you will have no protection against the vertebrae shifting sideways.

I now take you into an understanding of your spine and how to help yourself. Your spine is more than a bunch of small bones hanging together. It houses the cable network that transmits all the incoming and outgoing messages from your body to your brain. It is an upside down tree with connections to all the cables in the brain. In a sense, your spine, which contains your spinal cord, is your body's lifeline.

Spinal cord

Your spinal cord is about 18" long and slightly thicker than a pencil. It is suspended in the vertebral canal continuous with the medulla oblongata (the innermost part of the brain stem), until it reaches as low as the first or second lumbar vertebra. The cord has two swellings (enlargements) oval in section (in the cervical). It supplies the nerves to your upper extremity, to the arms, hands, and fingers, and the lumbar swelling is slightly smaller and supplies the nerves to your lower extremities, to your hips, thighs, legs, feet, and toes. Thirty-two pairs of spinal nerves are connected with the spinal cord.

THE SIGNIFICANCE OF YOUR SPINAL CORD

Each segment of your spinal cord can be likened to a small hamlet on a freeway or a main road. Each segment has its own existence and function to perform. Each segment sends messages along the freeway or road from its particular territory to the brain, the hamlet at the end of the road. From here all information, which now is coordinated, is sent back along this freeway or road. Injury to the cord may affect any or all of these functions.

The spinal nerves control your vitality and your health. They control your blood circulation, which is important to all bodily functions. You have blushed some moments during your life from embarrassment, or turned ashen when you were frightened. These were responses of your nervous system controlling the large blood vessels, which had shut down the small blood vessels completely. Just think about what can happen if a nerve in your your back is compressed and irritated by constant pressure, how it would influence the blood flow to the smaller vessels leading to your heart, stomach, or lungs? Disease could develop if the pressure is not removed. Heart attacks and strokes are attributable to pressures on the nerves influencing the blood vessels.

Take care of your spine. Keep the vertebrae supple. Keep your circulation free. This will improve your vitality and your health. Have your back examined periodically, not just your front. This way you will avoid sickness and unnecessary surgery.

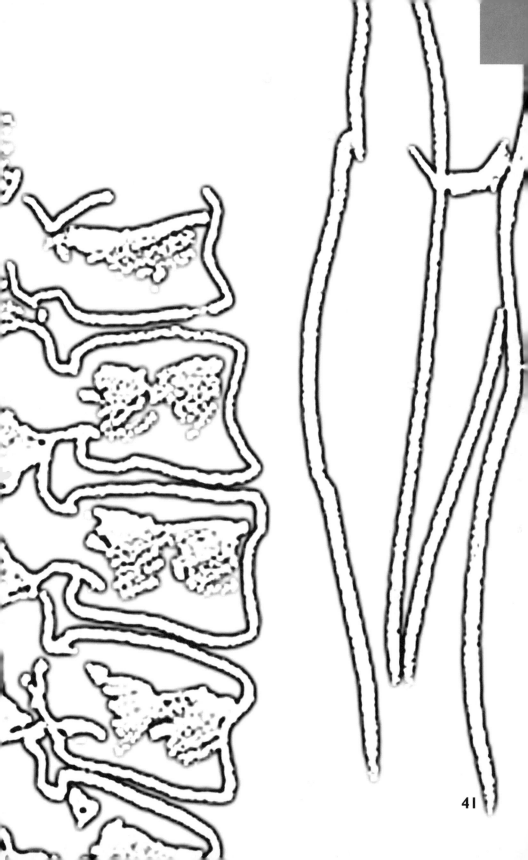

41

NOW TEST YOURSELF

(Please use a separate sheet of paper.)

1. What is compensation?

2. What is the meaning of "lesion"?

3. What is the motion to the muscles?

4. To remove pain, what procedures should you attempt?

5. Deep touch is felt through which fingers?

6. What is most important in healing?

7. What does your skin reflect?

CHAPTER 4:

UNDERSTANDING HOW TO HELP YOUR SPINE

Mankind was given definite problems
to solve, but also intelligence to
solve these problems.
Understanding attained through effort
And experience has a real value
In the revelation of the meanings
Behind these problems.

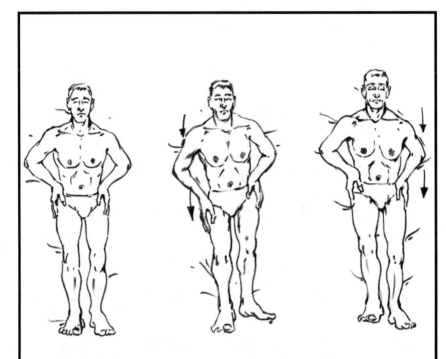

1. Lie in bed in the supine position, exercising the quadratus and psoas muscles.

2. Elevate your left hip by stretching the right quadratus and psoas muscles.

3. Now elevate your right hip by stretching the left quadratus and psoas muscles.

Pause and breathe normally.

Relax and repeat as long as you are feeling relaxed. Do this twice daily.

A Most Important Exercise

This exercise is for ladies who have pain during the menstrual cycle.

When my daughter had just begun her period, she was having pains. I gave her the following exercise.

1. Both knees flexed on the bed, sitting or lying down.
2. Both feet facing and touching one another, big toe to big toe, little toe to little toe.
3. Knees will remain wide apart.

This exercise will release the tension on the muscles on the pubis. She told all her friends who suffered from pains during the menstrual cycle.

If you find a painful area along the ligaments which border between your thighs and your lower abdominal muscles it will help to begin to massage them. This too will ease the menstrual pain. You may massage the trapezeus muscles on your shoulders close to your neck. And, if these pains exhaust you, massage your breast plate for a few moments; repeat several times.

To quicken your recovery from exhaustion or afternoon fatigue, take some thyme and make it into tea. Drink two or three cups during your period or whenever you feel tired or exhausted.

FOR MEN AND WOMEN BOTH: RELAXING THE PSOAS MUSCLE
Only the side affected should be relaxed. Begin:

1. Lie flat on a sofa or your bed.
2. Keep the leg on the unaffected side straight but relaxed.
3. Flex your leg on the affected side, while bringing it upward, forming the figure four.
4. Place the arch of the foot against the knee on the leg that is straight. Do not place the foot on the leg. That's a no-no!
5. With the hand on the straight leg side find the umbilicus.

45

6. Move your fingers slightly toward the flexed leg and press down on the muscles of your abdomen. Then release.

7. Press and release several minutes. After this, sit up, keeping the legs as they are.

8. Press on the flexed knee downward for a few seconds. Release and press again.

9. You may now get up.

YOU WILL HAVE HELPED YOURSELF A GREAT DEAL.

When your spine is in balance from your sacrum to the skull, its ability to do its work is at its maximum. Your spine will not need compensation to help it in its work. But your spine is seldom in a state of balance. To maintain balance, it is necessary to relearn old habits in standing, in sitting, and even in reclining.

But this is not all you will have to relearn. Exercise—an instrument in maintaining health—can be an instrument in creating injuries, temporary and permanent. These must also become important considerations each time you begin a form of exercise. For example: playing racquetball while healthy, tears muscle tissue and jars the joints in your body. Tennis tears the joints in your knees. Golf twists your back and your knees.

Your back must also be in equilibrium while having intimate relations. I have helped to remove pain in many of my patients who injured themselves during sexual activity. Knowledge in this area is limited or rarely explained by doctors.

Your were fashioned not for destruction but for life, to acquire wisdom, to experience love and the joy of peace and a harmonious existence by sharing yourself and others with you. You learn to balance your everyday existence and make compensations where needed—as does your spine.

When your spine is functioning perfectly in the upright position or posture then the center of gravity runs through the center of your spine, called the midline. In order to know how a lesion occurs in your spine, keep this midline in your mind. Close your eyes and visualize a fine "light thread" running from your head down to the tip of your sacrum. Having done this, remember that any fixed deviation from this midline in any direction by one or more vertebrae is a lesion or a subluxation on the mechanics of your spine, and your body will have to compensate for it.

What is "compensation"? It is a process by which your body attempts to maintain balance or equilibrium. Compensation is only needed when something needs to be adjusted or corrected. Stress in your body will spread until it is completely masked or until the body breaks down. This applies to your back as well as to the various systems in your body, not excluding your mind and your emotions.

Each time you stand up or do anything in the standing position, your human machine, your body, must compensate for being in the upright posture. Your muscles perform a very important role in maintaining equilibrium, which is compensation for your body's state of imbalance and distortion.

Compensation extends into all vital and mental processes. Your body is a whole, composite structure, and it functions in harmony with all its various systems. When stress occurs anywhere in your body's systems, lesion or lesions will occur, and compensation begins in order to adjust that imbalance.

You have undoubtedly heard your friends say to you, or you may have said it to your friends, "I had a pain just like this a week ago," "a month ago," or "the other day." This is not true. No person has the "like this" pain. Similar pain, yes. Patients have told me, "Doctor, I have the same pain I had the last time I saw you." My reply was, "No human being can remember pain precisely how he experienced it and felt it and recall it consciously, let alone ascribe this present pain exactly the same degree and intensity. Memory plays tricks on the conscious mind. Each lesion carries its own peculiar character at this new moment of distortion or imbalance. Your pain is similar, but not the same."

Familiarity often breeds contempt, but not always. There is great wisdom in seeking a familiarity as it relates to your health. You must look for differences in your conclusions as to what has caused your problem, what the problem is, and how to maintain your health in the best way. This is a basic tenet of attaining wisdom regarding your health.

There is a language to health
and a language to disease
He that wishes to heal
needs to know both
in order that he may gain
an insight into the ways
help may be rendered.

Every word has a root in another word, like a sapling from a tree. So, too, the word lesion, whose meaning is derived from the Latin word laesio, meaning injury. Injury means any pathological or traumatic condition that disrupts healthy functioning of the body or one of its organs or its parts, or simply anything that is wrong with the body.

Your body was born with your individual capacity to handle various types of stresses, weights or loads it can carry. You may carry your stresses better than others, or you may be able to carry two people on your back, while your friends may be able to carry none. You may be able to worry less than someone else, or you may worry more than your friends.

Remember that anything that interferes with your back's health in any way or any one of its segments will eventually cause it to suffer. The spinal cord will be denied its ability to function properly in the area or segment involved, not just nutritionally, from the weblike blood vessels that surround the cord, but in its ability to put out physical nerve impulses. The nerve trunk that supplies the muscles of your joints supplies as well the muscles that move the joints and the skin over the muscles where they insert. Therefore, you feel pain to the touch in particular joints in your body. Palative treatment of any chronic injury, such as by massage or by deep, steady pressure on the nerves, will only fatigue the nerve rather than remove the cause.

Any motion or movement is a form of stimulation to the muscles. In your attempt to remove pain or discomfort, you should apply deep, slow motion, relaxing the soft tissue and, in the process, remove stagnant toxic fluids which have been irritating your nerves and your muscles. This will relax the tissues.

Have you looked at your hands lately? What have you seen? Do you say to yourself, "Are they ugly?" or "Are they nice?" Are they young-looking, or are they old and wrinkled? Are they callused or smooth? How were they when they were young; how are they now? Have they done good work? Have they uplifted someone? Or, have they been raised to strike someone? Have they caressed or have they harassed? Have they held another hand in love? Or, have they pushed away someone who wished to love? All these are your hands, but it is the hand of Life that makes you able to do all of these and keeps you going, even when your mind fails you.

Your hands receive sensations from your epicritic (light touch that determines accurately fine variations in temperatures and touch) and deep sensibilities that are turned into definite perceptions, which in turn are perceived as mental impressions of the object you touch. The same things happen when your doctor touches you. The doctor conceives an idea about your condition. His examination may indicate different conditions in the tissues he examines such that he determines the kind of problem in evidence. If you are sensitive enough, you may come to the same conclusions through self-examination. You will be aware of soggy or swollen tissue, but only your doctor will be aware of tissue that is without good tone quality as a result of your thyroid underfunctioning; paralyzed, or underdeveloped, or damaged tissue; loss of tissue due to disuse; tissue depressed due to drugs; or damaged or toxic tissue from infection or fatigue. In these your doctor has more experience. Don't give up; always be aware of your body.

These different concepts that you and especially your doctor receive through touch are as real to the hands as is sound to the ear and color to the eye. It takes time to develop the skill in order to detect these differences. Your doctor will not talk while examining you. Listen to what his hands reveal about you.

Bones are conductors of sound. The doctor has developed a sensitivity to the

• •

sounds your body makes under his hand or his finger. You have the same ability to develop your "hearing" through your hands. Sound is conducted to the brain by vibration of the molecules that hit not just your ear, but your entire body. Your feet sense the rhythm of music or the sound traveling through the ground or water long before your ears are involved. To hear these vibrations, all you have to do is focus your attention on your body.

There are two distinct types of touch: "light" touch and "deep." Light touch is performed by the use of epicritic sensibility. This touch is a fine discrimination between heat and coldness of the tissue or the temperature of the body. This sensibility exists in your skin only. When you wish to determine the temperature of a joint or the body, place your entire palm on the surface you wish to examine, e.g., a pain in your abdomen, foot, or hand.

Deep touch combs the deep nerve terminals and your muscles. Deep touch is a learned ability and something you should not attempt on yourself or allow just anyone to do to you, especially if they are not qualified. Masseuses are not trained to determine causes and methods of treatment. When in doubt, seek the advice your doctor can provide. Deep touch is usually felt through the first phalanx of your thumb and the first and second fingers. To examine the back, as well as the buttock and around the hip, deep touch is to be used.

Feeling is not poking. Never poke yourself or anyone else or let anyone do that to you. Whenever you examine yourself, be careful to find only what is actually there and not what you imagine should be there or what you wish to be there. Do not fool yourself. Read further in this book and consult your doctor.

Stop for the moment to consider how you use your hands. You can help heal or kill by the same hand. No one has resurrected the one who was killed by his hand or by his tongue. Let no one feel the weight of your hand or tongue, except for loving-kindness or to restore life.

To practice how to feel with your hands, so that you may know how your body feels when healthy and when in a state of disease, close your eyes and your mouth and see what your hands will see (discover). Do this with both hands, exchanging hands as you go along in this book. You will be shown how you can help yourself in minor conditions, but not when major conditions affect you. But remember, should you find a minor condition, do not fix it until you are sure that it is minor. It is important to first refer to the material discussed in later chapters. Then, when you're sure, proceed to help yourself.

There is nothing more important in the art of healing than the proper diagnosis, for diagnosis is a process in finding what physical state or physiological condition your body is in. Your doctor has taken much time to learn how to help you. If you wish to be of help to yourself, you must spend many hours to know your own body through reading, observation, and by taking an interest in yourself. In diagnosis, your doctor uses curiosity, imagination, confidence, and perseverance to arrive at a proper and correct diagnosis. Your physical examination by yourself or your physician depends entirely upon the senses. Your physician should be able to make a practical diagnosis of your condition without the aid of gadgets or chemical tests or x-rays. The hands of your doctor and his/her judgment are the most valued material possessions. He should protect them, and so should you protect your hands and develop your judgment. Always be observant, especially about your health. Your doctor's first impression upon meeting you will not be from your medical condition but from your facial expression, and from the anxiety your body exhibits from the pain it is experiencing. He will draw his conclusions also from the color of your skin, how you carry yourself, how you walk, what state your body is in terms of its posture (side-bent, forward bent, which may indicate lumbago, sciatica, a strain or strains, gall bladder pain, or kidney stones), and so forth.

Your skin reflects the tension of your nerves. You can develop what is known as neurodermatitis, an itching, because you are nervous about something. The cure? Reduce tension. Do not scratch these areas or you might break the skin. Vitamin B complex may help to control tension. Follow the exercises given in the latter part of the book, but now here is one that will help you to release your tension. Tension wears down your adrenal glands and you may develop problems with low blood sugar, which in turn causes nerve tension. Now you are going around in circles. To help yourself, eat a balanced meal. Exercise to relax. Do this exercise regularly.

1. Find your abdomen.

2. Place the flat pads of your fingers around the navel.

3. Gently massage the reflex area for about 60 seconds. This will relax you.

I want you to understand that daily exercise is essential to proper metabolism. Exercise will keep your blood sugar from skipping around; it will remain more even and improve your vitality. Help yourself to progress; keep yourself on the move; be encouraged in your efforts; drive ahead with zeal; but help someone else along on their quest while you are at yours.

Have you ever walked on the street or in a park, or in a concert hall or a ball game, and tried to find out what is wrong with the person who is ahead of you? Try it. It will teach you to be observant and develop empathy for your fellow human beings. There is always someone who is studying you, wherever you are. This way others sharpen their skills of observation. You become the object from which they have learned. You become their teacher at the same time. Once, when my late wife and I attended the Academy Awards, Raquel Welch was on stage. As she walked away, I turned to my wife and said, "Look. She has a slight problem walking." My wife replied, "Only you would notice her walk; everyone else is looking at her breasts."

Look in the mirror when you are alone. Observe how your pelvis is positioned, whether it is in rotation, whether it is forward or backward in tilt. Look for your spine's curvatures. Pay attention to your lumbar curve and the compensations your shoulders make—which is higher, which is lower—and how your head tilts. Look for discoloration of your skin, for moles, for fatty tumors, or anything that may be suspicious. Move your spine, test your flexibility or find your rigidity, and make note of these. Develop the skill of observation every chance you have.

The juncture of your neck, including your upper back below your shoulder blades (the scapulae), is a very important area of your back. It is vulnerable to trauma more than any other area of your spine. This area is subject to stresses from your constant compensation as your lower spine base is tilted. Here your major nerve plexus (brachial) nourishes your arms, your hands, and your fingers. The vasomotor nerves, which supply your entire head, arms, heart, and lungs, come from this area, and the autoprotective apparatus, which consists of the pituitary, thyroid, and adrenals, receive part of the nerve supply from this area. This area is exposed to direct strain from physical activity and will always be congested and will always be in muscular contractions.

Human beings lose their fear of the hand when the touch feels good, when the hand is placed from the lower part of the neck (cervical spine) to the (fifth thoracic) lower scapula. Keep the palm of your hand in contact with the body while you hold the muscles between your thumb and finger, and you will note how fast this will relax you and those whom your hand touches. Can you stretch forth your hand against any man and not be found guilty before the Creator? Can you?

Each day, 2 to 3 times during the day, dangle your body from an overhead bar. Stretch your muscles. Dangling is the key. Your back must be supple at all times.

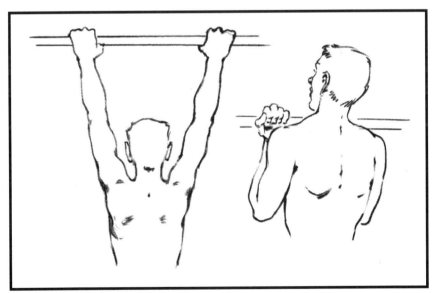

Chinning: Developing strength in your arms

CHAPTER 5 EXAMINATION

NOW TEST YOURSELF

(Please use a separate sheet of paper.)

1. How should an injury in your back be evaluated?

2. Can a maladjustment be seen on an x-ray?

3. What is a signal that you have a problem in a joint?

4. What is a swelling?

5. When do muscles pull unequally?

6. What are the most important characteristics of an acute lesion?

7. What is soft tissue?

8. Should you immobilize a joint?

9. What is the purpose of synovial fluid?

10. What is the importance of the sound of a "pop"?

11. What intervertebral fragments do not contain lymphatics, veins, arteries, branches of the cerebrospinal and sympathetic nerves?

12. On what does the health of any organ depend?

CHAPTER 5:

SPINAL LESIONS

The anatomy of the individual person
is the physical and spiritual wholeness
as related to the stresses and the
harmony between its inner parts and
their outward expressions
either as tranquility or disease.

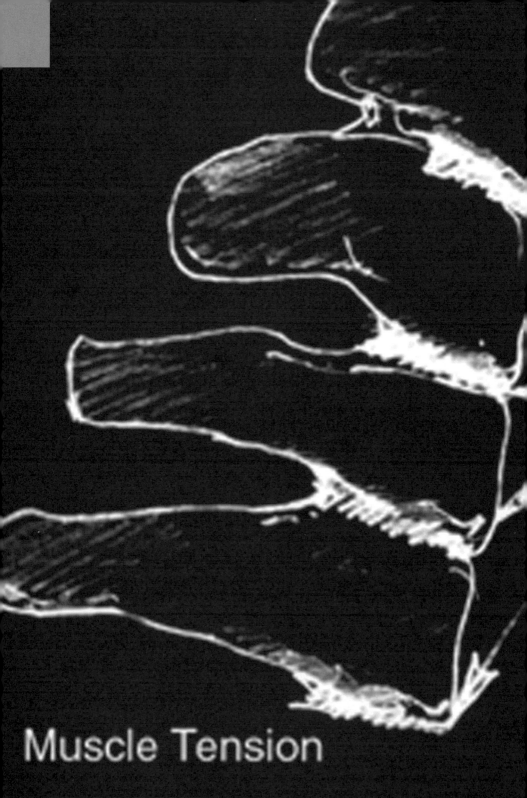

Muscle Tension

How often have you said, "Doctor, my back is out, can you help me?" What did you mean by it? You meant that you have a backache somewhere in a segment of your spine. (Your spinal cord after an injury will act independently from your brain. It performs many functions which are dependent only on the cord.) When the bones in your back are maladjusted, the symptoms they create may be severe; you will usually find changes in the tissues around the site where two vertebrae meet. When you apply pressure on the muscles, these will give you pain. Usually the muscle becomes hard; motion is diminished in the joint affected. Do these show up on an x-ray? No, but your doctor's hands should be able to detect them. You will know they exist because you are experiencing the pain.

You will notice that around the affected joint there will be varying masses of swollen and sometimes congested tissue. This should signal a problem, as this lesion must have been present for some days or even weeks. By now the area has become fibrotic, having a hardened texture in appearance and to the touch, adding to the size of the bone.

An injury between two vertebrae is a disturbed relationship, just like that between two persons, and you should not ignore it. This disturbed relationship can result from unequal muscle pull or shortened ligaments that hold your individual vertebrae together. One thing you should keep in mind is that your bones do not of themselves assume either a normal or abnormal position. Each vertebra shape is designed to fit together in their proper order. Therefore, upon movement of your spine, every single vertebra will return to its normal position if possible.

What will make your back go out of alignment, as many of my patients used to refer to their back pains? My answer was that vertebrae can be thrown out of their normal relations by trauma, such as a simple blow; by some disturbance in the ligaments; by unequal muscle pull, which may be sudden or prolonged over a period of time; by disease of the joints or the vertebrae themselves; by excessive pressures; or by swellings. In all cases, your vertebrae and ligaments are only passive contributors. Swelling is a biochemical activity. Your muscles do not pull unequally or abnormally except when under some adverse influence. Thus it is important to determine the cause of the lesion, but equally important not to merely guess at the cause.

You might have used the terms "acute" or "chronic" to describe a condition because of the length of time it has existed. Pain and swelling indicate an acute lesion to which your body's reaction is to limit movement as a defense against the injury.

The two most important characteristics for you to be aware of should you have chronic spinal injury are increased connective tissue and limited mobility. As your lesions become chronic—not acute—the swelling and pain also diminish. Connective tissue increases and motion in the joint diminishes. The lesion can be felt but does not cause trouble. It may appear to be dormant, but lesions are never dormant, at least I have never seen them in my many years of practice. During this quiescent state, changes take place that may eventually cause problems.

There is no distinct line that anyone can draw between an acute and a chronic lesion. Remember, to the degree swelling and pain subside, tissue increases and your mobility diminishes. Now the lesion qualifies as chronic.

You have been taught that bones are hard, but this is not so. Your normal living bone is plastic. The normal disc between your vertebrae is easily compressed under stress, and this compression will cause the disc's nutrition to become diminished and the disc to become deformed. I am sure you have felt a miraculous relief as soon as slight tension has been released and slight mobility established in your back or in a joint. This comes about by returning nourishment to the affected area. In an older person, where the bones seemingly have fused together ("ankylosed") relief can be felt when enough space is created between the surfaces to restore even a miniscule amount of mobility.

TREATMENT OF SOFT TISSUE

Muscle tissue remembers all movements from the time of formation of the embryo in the womb. These muscles will resume activity if assisted early enough after injury.

Soft tissue always possesses a "feel" that indicates the state of its health or pathology. On your back it will indicate which segment of your spine is affected. It is difficult for you to differentiate between healthy or pathological tissue except by the pain you experience. You may try to stretch and relax these muscles, but unless you free, by mobilizing the vertebra, the soft tissue, the organs that are supplied by the nerves and blood vessels will not benefit. At this point you should seek professional help.

The great good you derive from mobilization is the increased circulation of your spinal cord and the increased output of the nerves to the organs that they supply. Your spinal cord is filled with spinal fluid, an indicator of health or sickness. The reason you must never immobilize a joint is that it is difficult to normalize, and your discomfort will increase as the joint becomes frozen. I have found in my practice that when spinal segments of the upper back were locked or in a frozen state, the patient suffered a bout of pneumonia, pleurisy, gall bladder problems, or heart problems. Whenever I was able to give relief by an adjustment at the nerve center of the spinal segment, I helped my patient's recovery.

It is imperative for you to maintain mobility in each and every segment of your spine in order to maintain health. I have helped to relieve asthma attacks and bronchial pneumonia by adjusting the upper back. Then the supportive treatment (e.g., medications prescribed by a doctor) was effective.

What you should keep in mind is that all corrections have one end, which is to normalize the physiological functioning of deep structures within the body.

JOINTS AND "POP"

I have been asked by my patients, "What is that 'pop' sound I hear when I turn or when I exercise?" Here is my explanation: The surfaces of the joints in your body are separated constantly by synovial fluid. This fluid keeps the surfaces of your joints lubricated, like the oil on the hinges of a door to prevent it from squeaking and the oil in your car to prevent the pistons from causing your engine to burn out. The synovial fluid functions the same way by preventing the destruction of your joints.

When a joint such as your knee is held under constant tension by muscles which are in a state of contraction, the surface that carries the weight tends to become dry. This dryness is the first stage of joint pathology. Normal joints can be separated to produce a popping sound without injuring the ligaments. The joints that hold the synovial fluids are closed cavities, and the fluid in them flushes the surfaces with beneficial effect. When a synovial joint is separated, the popping sound is the same whether it is a vertebral joint or the knee.

It is good for you to remember that with the exception of the first atlas and second cervical and the sacral, each intervertebral foramen (opening) contains lymphatics, veins, arteries, the branches of the cerebrospinal and sympathetic nerves. Besides these, there is a great amount of tissue that is often in a tense state from the abnormal positions of the vertebrae or are thickened as a result of mechanical or toxic irritations. No wonder that such important changes take place as a result of lesions in the intervertebral joints and surfaces! Remember that the neck is to be respected. Avoid traumatizing it. Do not twist your neck, as in wrestling, and do not carry heavy objects on your neck, head, or shoulders.

The fact is that the health of any of your organs depends upon the nerve and blood supply they receive. So, too, your life depends upon how you feel: the kind of thoughts you are thinking, the kind of feelings you either express or hide from yourself, whether you keep the lifeline open between your life and the life of others and the All Life that surrounds us. Therefore, the health of the nerves depends upon how free they are from obstruction. Each segment of your spine must be kept free from obstructing the nerves that emerge from the spinal cord.

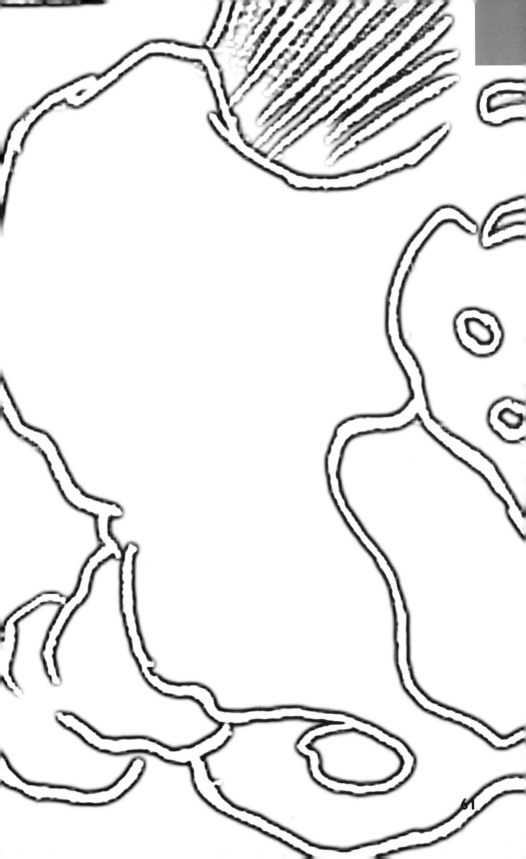

61

CHAPTER 6 EXAMINATION

NOW TEST YOURSELF

(Please use a separate sheet of paper.)

1. What is a correction?

2. What does "thrust" convey?

3. What is a "tap"?

4. What factors control nutrition?

5. How do you normalize blood flow?

6. Where does physiological change begin?

7. What is the difference between yourself and an infant?

8. How old are you?

9. What is motility?

10. Does old tissue respond to treatment?

11. What two lesions are your sacroiliac subject to?

12. When do you produce a sacroiliac lesion?

13. What is the sacred bone associated with?

CHAPTER 6:

CORRECTING A LESION

Always complete your task
Else
a part of you will never rest
For in your task your very
Self
is found!

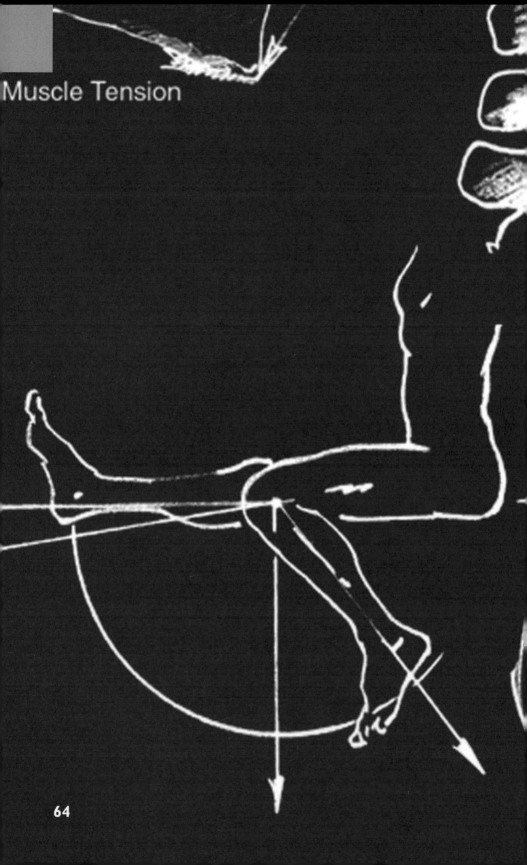

Muscle Tension

"**A**djustment" to many people means the "cracking" of bones, but its actual meaning is the act of correction or manipulation of the misaligned articulations between two vertebral segments or group of articulating segments, which are called lesions.

Adjustments are something we all make in life. We adjust to a new situation, a new home, a new job, a new companion, new foods, a new car, and new ideas. Adjustment implies a sense of well being, a kind of harmony, a feeling of contentment, a feeling of being satisfied. To adjust your back is therefore a process of restoring the health to your spine or to a joint in your body.

Never allow anyone to make a sudden thrusting movement to your back or on any one joint. This kind of sudden push can seem violent, and with it comes fear, tension, and pains.

Only minimum force or touch is required to correct a lesion. Minimum force yields maximum results—that is nature's way of doing things. If your doctor's touch is light you will not experience any pain.

Make sure not to tense your body while getting an adjustment. Do not flinch, because flinching causes tension, which is a barrier to returning the joints to normal. Neither you nor your doctor should overlook tension or soreness in your muscles. Do not cause more irritation to them through massage. If you need to slow down the reflexes in your muscles before you are adjusted, have your doctor prescribe a mild sedative.

You are responsible for your health, not just by what you eat but through your fears, your hopes, your faith, your anger, and the history you write upon your body and mind at each moment you move and breathe. Good health requires good nutrition. Your nutrition is controlled by two main factors. First, you must have good nerve supply to your digestive system. To do this, you must keep the nerves free from impingement on your spine. Second, you must have good blood circulation throughout your body. Anything that impedes the nerve supply and circulation will interfere with your body's ability to gain the full benefit from your food intake.

When you are in a horizontal position, your heart does not experience the strain of lifting a great load. If you exercise in this position, your heart will have very little cause for heart failure, and there will be sufficient blood flow throughout your body. When you are in an upright position working all day, your brain, which is above your heart, tends to become slightly anemic. This causes the brain to function somewhat slower than when you are in the horizontal position. Your eyes and ears are also affected. In fact, all structures above your heart in the erect-upright position are affected, including the upper part of your lungs.

What happens to the region below your heart? These areas become congested, and the heart becomes vulnerable to a breakdown due to overwork. When you go to sleep and try to read, the heart works hard to equalize the blood flow in your body. Before you go to sleep it would help your heart to hang the upper part of your body over your bed, letting your shoulders, arms, and head hang down for 60 seconds. This helps the heart to equalize the blood in your body. In addition, your sinuses will unclog, your breathing improve, and, if you have a sinus headache, it will lessen. During the day your intestines, stomach, and all your organs press downward on your bladder. This overhang will help in their normalization as well. Before you do this exercise, make sure that you do not hang from your waist down. That would be unwise; you may tip over. Only your head, arms, and shoulders should hang over the bed. Your body below your shoulder blades must remains on the bed.

SECOND YOUTH

Here I am concerned with the physical and degenerative changes in the body that lead to senility and other mental aberrations. (I have learned that youth is a state that exists between the eyes and not below it.) It is important to remember that physiological change begins on the cellular level, where the cell plasma is slowly replaced by connective tissue, which degenerates with age. When you are very young, the cells in your body have an abundance of protoplasm; with age, the cells lose protoplasm and begin to thicken.

The difference between you as an infant and you at your present age is the quality and quantity of your cytoplasm, cell plasma, and connective tissue. When you were a child, the tissue in your body was soft and elastic; now your tissues are less elastic and they may become hard and rigid. The age of your cells is determined by their physical condition and not by the years they have been in your body (that is, your chronological age).

You are as old as the condition of your tissues. They hold your body together, supporting your blood vessels, nerves, organs, and lymphatics. Connective tissues attach your bones from your toes to the knees, hips, arms, and fingers. All these tissues are well supplied with nerves.

Keep in mind that the main characteristic of these tissues is that they eventually become shortened, causing the loss of vitality in the cell. When your arteries thicken, good circulation is impeded; and when connective tissue shortens and thickens around your joints, your mobility is affected, so you move slowly and with difficulty. If they thicken around an organ, like a lung or the liver, their motility is affected. Motility is the independent movement of an organ within the body. Each organ is capable of independent movement—each nerve has its own nerve supply as each blood vessel has its own blood and nerve supply.

Keep your body youthful by not abusing it through overwork, stress, poor nutrition, and forceful exercise. Never allow your mind to rule your body. Your mind is dependent upon keeping your connective tissues' health so that it will send a constant supply of blood to your brain, ensuring that new brain cells will develop.

SO YOU THINK THERE IS NO HELP

Power leads to health
Powerlessness leads to disease
Be it in body or mind
Regardless of physical age.

Because you are advanced in years, does this mean you can get no relief if you have a hardened lesion in your back? Not at all! I have helped people who were more than 90 years old. You must discard the erroneous notion that because of your age you cannot be helped. I assure you, based on my experience, old tissue responds to treatment quicker than tissue that is more elastic and much younger.

What needs to be done is to increase nutrition into the area to reduce the rigidity. Relief is given by relaxing the rigid tissue and encouraging the flow of vital fluids into the area. This permits cells that can break down tissues that have hardened to be brought into the area, keeping the toxins contained.

When the tissue is in an acute state, you must treat it gently. When the inflammation or irritability subsides, treatment can be more forceful, so that elasticity may be increased and healing can begin. When a joint in your spine becomes maladjusted, or it "goes out," it will be held in that position by the inflamed, now abnormal soft tissue tension. At this stage you should seek help from your doctor who will release the joints to normalize the maladjusted areas. Your joints will have limited mobility, and must be released by stretching first.

Rule #1: Remember, if you find that the tissue around your joints is not very rigid, gentle stretching will be sufficient.

Rule #2: If your tissue around the joint is very tough or appears to be brittle (that is, if it has lost its elasticity), the tap method will break down the tissue quickly and permit nourishment to reach the cells in that area.

Keep this in mind: Motion is the speech of life in the universe. If you allow yourself to become inactive, exposing yourself to worry, tension, boredom, and general debility, your joints will become stiff and immobile. Create motion in your joints daily—even if you move only a little. If you need assistance, ask someone to help you. Each day move your joints a bit further. If you hips are tight, lie down on your back, then have someone rotate your feet in both directions. Do both rotations, one foot at a time or simultaneously, making sure that both toes point in or out at the same time. Next, move the knees by flexing them. Then, rotate the feet. Your knees must be flexed individually and gently without pressure. Lastly, make a circular motion with your feet.

Now do the following:

1. Sit comfortably on your bed, cross one ankle over one knee, and press the knee of the crossed leg down. This will release pain and discomfort in your hips and legs. If you have arthritic pain, this is especially helpful because it slows down the degeneration in your joints.

2. Exercise your shoulders by making circular movements in both directions with your arms extended. If you are not able to move your arms or hold them up, have someone move them for you. Be sure to move your elbows and your wrists.

Remember: Exercise. Increase your circulation. Increase your fluid intake. Movement and water hydration are what keep you going.

SACROILIAC JOINT

Your sacroiliac, like all joints, is subject to two lesions (injuries). The first is caused by strain and the second is caused by one side of the joint moving past its limit and locking in that position. To repair the first requires time, rest, and/or treatment; whereas the second can be easily corrected. This is due to the fact that inside ligaments—those that face the inside of your body—are very weak in comparison to those outside (facing the skin). Those ligaments facing the skin are easy to separate from the joint through stress or injury.

The majority of sacroiliac injuries are produced when the legs are apart or one of your feet is firmly on the ground while your body is turned away from it, which can happen while playing golf. When you stand on one leg too long, for example, or put your pants on while standing on one foot, you stretch one side of your ligaments by putting all your weight on one side. This action will cause you to be off balance. One side was meant to carry only half of your weight!

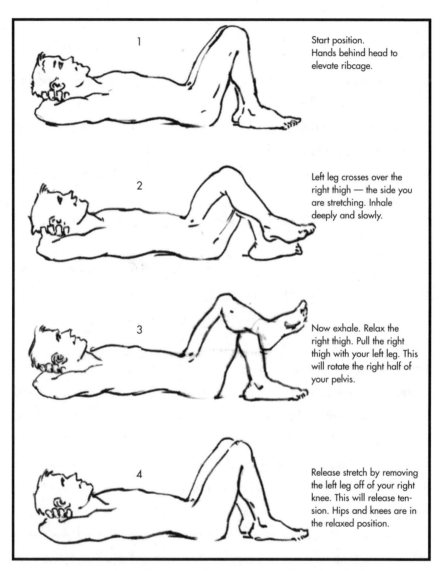

1 Start position.
Hands behind head to
elevate ribcage.

2 Left leg crosses over the
right thigh — the side you
are stretching. Inhale
deeply and slowly.

3 Now exhale. Relax the
right thigh. Pull the right
thigh with your left leg. This
will rotate the right half of
your pelvis.

4 Release stretch by removing
the left leg off of your right
knee. This will release tension. Hips and knees are in
the relaxed position.

Exercise for Quadratus Lumbar Muscle

Your sacroiliac joint is held together by ligaments that are connective tissue and are prone to injury. Your job is to minimize your chances of injuring yourself. I am sure you do not wish to walk bent over from your sacrum or your "sacred bone," another name for the sacroiliac, the foundation of your spine. This sacred bone is associated with disabilities of the back, or with our ability to make love, encompassing our greatest pleasures and our greatest pains.

Remember, tension over your sacrum in time will reduce motion, just like any other joint in your body, and a stiff joint can become arthritic. Tension and pressure affect the circulation in the muscles and the nerves that pass through them resulting in an undernourished joint.

You can help yourself by lying down on your back and pulling your knees up toward your chest. Grasp them with both hands and push your knees away from your hands as hard as you can. This will loosen your back muscles as well as your hamstrings. The hardest working muscles will relax first. Whenever you strain your back while bending or twisting, the muscles involved are the quadratus lumborum and the psoas muscles. In front of the quadratus muscle are the kidneys, the psoas muscles, and the diaphragm, which affects respiration. The muscle begins in the ilio-lumbar ligament. Near the crest of your ilia it is connected to the lower rib and the upper four lumbar vertebrae.

If you hurt yourself and have difficulty walking, do the following: Press your hands inward below your ribs, over your love handles. At the same time, press downward. This will enable you to bypass your lumbar spine as it relaxes the muscle and keeps pain to a minimum, and you will be able to walk slowly. Keep your head up and take slow, deep breaths while you walk. Holding your head up relieves pressure in the low back.

* *

This is another exercise for releasing these muscles through stretching:

1. Lie on your back, and place your hands behind your head This will elevate your ribcage.

2. Pull your knees up, with your feet on the bed or floor.

3. Cross your leg over the knee on the affected side.

4. Inhale and hold your breath as you pull with your leg the knee on the affected side. This will rotate your pelvis and release the tension and the pain by lengthening the muscles that have shortened due to strain.

5. Slowly bring your legs back to the starting position. Exhale and relax.

6. Uncross your leg. Do this exercise slowly a couple of times.

7. DO NOT DO THIS ON THE SIDE THAT IS NOT AFFECTED. Remember this, or you will risk further injury.

In the hearts of all the living
Hope and faith are often mixed
With doubt, love and disappointment
Expectations and bitterness

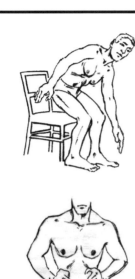

Muscle Strain — Quadratus — is often affected by bending or twisting.

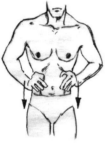

If you have pain in your Quadratus lumbar muscle and you are not able to walk, press your hands inward and downward. This will bypass your lumbar spine and you will be able to walk slowly.

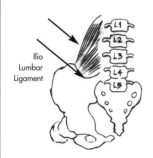

Ilio
Lumbar
Ligament

L1
L2
L3
L4
L5

Quadratus Lumborum Muscle as seen from the front.

CHAPTER 7 EXAMINATION

NOW TEST YOURSELF

(Please use a separate sheet of paper.)

1. Who is responsible for taking care of you?

2. What four conditions in the self-examination should you be aware of?

3. What kind of motion is desired in the sacroiliac joint?

4. What causes tension?

5. What does it mean if you have a lesion in your sacroiliac?

6. When are x-rays indicated?

7. Pain in front of the hip area indicates what?

8. Pain in the back of the hip area indicates what?

9. What kind of joint is the hip?

10. What are the symptoms from your hip related to?

CHAPTER 7:

SELF-EXAMINATION

Accept the evil that exists inside of you
And that which is good
Accept the good and the evil
Which exists outside of you
For between these
Lies the narrow road of your life.

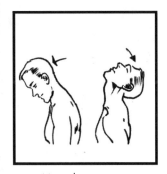

Normal movements

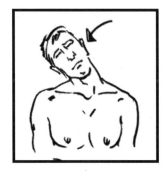

Normal range

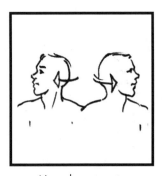

Normal movements

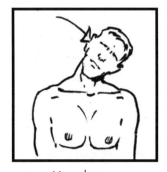

Normal range

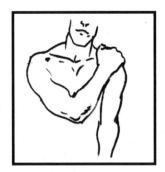

Test for internal rotation

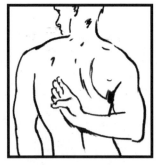

Internal rotation

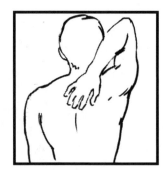

External rotation

*These are the normal tests of range-of-motion that
you can perform on yourself for the head and neck and the
movements of your arms.*

G o to a mirror. Look at yourself with critical eyes. See how you walk.

1. Notice if your pelvic area moves in a rhythmic pattern.
2. Does your pelvis jerk? If it does, notice to which side. Write it down. A jerking pelvis indicates that you have a problem on that side.
3. Do you limp on one side or the other?
4. Are your steps the same length at all times?
5. Do your toes point at the same angle?
6. Are your ankles bent inward or outward?
7. Do you have flat feet; or are they normal and healthy?
8. Check to see if you shift your weight from one foot to the other. Are your sacroiliacs tender to the touch?
9. Look at your general posture. Do you carry yourself fairly straight and comfortably; or are you bent over, with a dowager hump or a curve in your upper back?
10. Which leg appears shorter to you? It is possible that the inside muscle of the pelvis is affected and is pulled up? This gives the appearance of a short leg.

Why should you observe all of this? To avoid problems, you should know your body and know how to take care of it. Your doctor cannot take care of you minute-by-minute. You are always responsible for yourself.

HOW TO AVOID A RISING TEMPER THAT LEADS TO BLOOD PRESSURE ELEVATION

When your mind becomes tranquil, you have reached the starting gate in a constructive journey. If you allow your life to restore a state of tranquility to your mind, it will be protected from disruptive forces.

You can do something daily to help yourself and your body. Your face contains reflexes or points that can help to bring calm. Your neck also has reflexes that will help you; this is the case as well with the back of your head, a place you sel-

∙∙

dom see except when you look into a mirror. You can make use of these reflex areas, called Derma tomes, to help calm you down.

1. Between the eyebrows, at the roof of your nose, is a reflex center. Apply firm pressure with your carpal tunnel (the base of your hand where it joins your forearm) or your thumb for 45-60 seconds, two to three times a day.

2. Now feel your thyroid cartilage, your Adam's apple. Move your finger to one side over the skin covering it. Squeeze the skin between your finger or the nails of your forefinger and thumb for 20 seconds on each side of your neck. Do this two to three times a day.

3. Next, move your fingers behind your head at the juncture of your neck and shoulders. Apply a circular motion from left to right. This will reduce the power of a bad temper. You also will experience a relaxed feeling when you massage your forearms or your lower legs. Keep doing this; it will help calm you down. This is much more civil than breaking furniture or dishes or using some one as a punching bag.

While your adrenaline helps you to cope with stress, an excess can trigger an adverse reaction.

You can also do more physical exercise: run in place, go for a walk, do calisthenics. Exercise during the day and especially before coming home after work.

TOUCHING YOURSELF

If you develop a low back problem, do a self-examination to determine whether to seek medical aid from your M.D. or your D.C. There are certain conditions you should be aware of, and these are the same conditions your doctor will note when he or she examines you. Consider these points when you touch the sacroiliac area or joint:

1. The tension of your ligaments

2. How much mobility there is in the joint; or the lack of mobility

3. How tender the joint is to your touch

Your doctor will determine the position or the asymmetry of your joint.

Remember that you must avoid stretching your sacroiliac joint or causing additional strain on the ligaments in this area. It is quite difficult to treat a joint that has been stretched due to an accident, massage, during diagnosis, by traction treatment, or during weight lifting. A normal joint has equal mobility on both sides; an abnormal joint will be the least mobile where tense ligaments are present.

The lumbar vertebrae must always be checked for muscular, ligamentous, and fascia shortening, also for tension, to determine how much mobility you have in the lumbars, how tender the lumbars are. As you age, the character of your sacroiliac changes with you. If there is a swelling in this joint, mobility will be affected.

What causes tenderness? As a rule, tension in your ligaments, trauma to the joint, an asymmetrical joint called subluxation, arthritis, infection, or all of the above. You may also be hypersensitive in the area. This may come from your lower lumbar vertebrae or from the viscera in the pelvis; however, these are not considered a true tenderness.

Your bones are plastic, and they become distorted from stresses that are unequally applied or carried by them. These distortions are accepted as normal because of the body's ability to compensate, especially if the stress lasts over a period of time. This distortion is functionally normal and may never cause pain; nevertheless, it would be wise to correct the joint before it becomes set. I have seen gardeners who are completely distorted from bending, but they have no pain; their bodies have compensated. This distortion is functional, becoming chronic due to the failure to seek help.

When you seek treatment from your doctor, remember that by giving a name to a condition does not mean that it is a diagnosis. When you have a lesion in the sacroiliac, and the ankle, the knee, and/or the hip are slightly or grossly out of line, remem-

• •

ber that it will often reset itself normally and will at the same time correct other conditions when a slight tug is applied on the leg by a D.C. or a D.O. The doctor will want you to be totally relaxed, especially around your hip, telling you to keep your knees extended (straight) before he will execute the tug. The tug feels like something between a pull and a jerk. Please do not let a friend or member of your family or a masseur or a trainer in the gym perform this on you. Do not perform this on a child or on older people. It takes skill and years of practice.

The lesions in the sacroiliac often recur the same way in which they were first produced. Often you are not conscious of the circumstances that resulted in the problem. When a strain occurs in a balanced pelvis, this can easily be corrected. But when a lesion occurs in a pelvis distorted from some form of chronicity, you must look for the cause. This will take a long time to correct; therefore, keep these things in mind:

1. An unbalanced pelvis, which is caused by legs of unequal length that were not corrected, is a major predisposing factor.

2. The unbalanced pelvis will distort the bond and will weaken the joints. These will predispose you to a recurrence of the joint problem.

3. Strained ligaments, stretched ligaments, and fascia that are contracted are also important factors.

4. Mobility should be equal in both joints, but this is not always possible in certain occupations. If you happen to be a contortionist or dancer, where mobility in one sacroiliac joint is greater than in the other, this inequity is normal within limits.

5. If your lumbar area is rigid, this will predispose you to sacroiliac lesions. Therefore, if you can increase the mobility in the lumbar region, the strain on your sacroiliac will diminish.

6. Posture, especially bad posture, will put a constant strain on the sacroiliac and predispose you to a lesion.

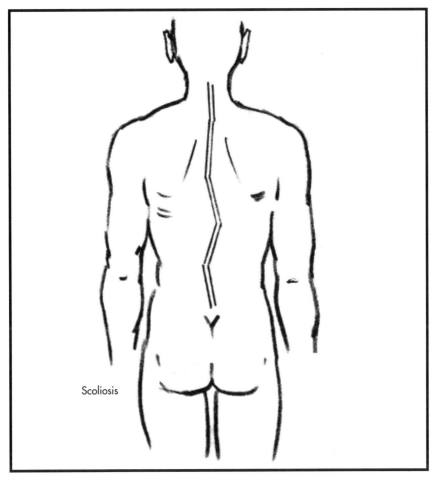

Scoliosis

Scoliosis should not stop you from normal living

THE HIP

There are times when your pelvis becomes so twisted that when you look at your feet, you will note that one foot is inverted (turned inward) and the other everted (turned outward). The head of the femur in the acetabulum, the opening in your pelvis, assumes the same position as the foot on the same side. The result is that it is "off center." This will interfere with the proper functions of the hip joint, and it will often cause

81

a vague general pain down the thigh, which could develop into a real hip pathology.

If for any reason you develop pain in the hip joint, it will usually be experienced as less than in other joints of your body because this joint is less sensitive to pain. If not, more serious conditions will be found upon close examination. It is important for you to be aware of this. Professional help should be sought for all hip joint pain.

If you develop arthritis in the hip joint, it will be due to strain on the ligaments and the fascia in the area. In this case, never allow the femur to be used as a lever in a correction of any sort.

The following considerations are important to your hip:

1. Simple inflammatory processes in your hip are rare. This is because your hip has a great range of motion. Motion is a sign of health in this area.

2. When there is pain and muscle spasms with splinting your hip joint, it will indicate a serious disease in the joint. Cancerous lesions are most common in the hip joint. This is probably due to the anatomical pull of the ligaments and surrounding capsule when the body assumes the erect position.

3. When such pain is experienced, x-rays should be taken. Do not delay!

4. If there was trauma to the hip, x-rays are indicated.

5. If a true hip joint pain develops within five years after a removal of a tumor or an exploratory operation, always take an x-ray or an MRI (Magnetic Resonance Imaging).

6. Pain in the anterior (front) hip area is most commonly caused by psoasitis (inflammation caused by stress or injury to the low back). This is produced by reflex via at least 18 abdominal pelvic and spinal factors. (The psoas muscles are the intra-abdominal muscles that cover the inner abdominal surface and become a part of the thigh.)

7. Pain in the posterior area (back) of the hip is due to sacroiliac strains or lesions, sciatic neuritis, and posterior myositis (that is, inflammation of a voluntary muscle).

8. Treatment in both cases should include the following: In psoasitis, stretching and

relaxing by manual traction, diathermy (heat treatment), or segmental block (cortisone injection into the lumbar disc). In the case of myositis, local treatment may include diathermy, stretching of the external rotators by internal rotation of the femur, and stretching of the hamstring musculature by straight leg raising, and other measures by intravenous injection.

9. Pain in the medial hip area is due to inflammation of the adductor muscles (muscles that draw toward the midline of your body). Adductor myositis is usually a result of weight shift from the side of involvement. Treatment is as noted above.

10. Pain on the side of your hip (lateral) may extend to the knee joint, which may be due to reflex and/or to trauma. Treatment is stretching and chiropractic treatment as noted in number 8 above.

IT IS IMPORTANT TO REMEMBER THE FOLLOWING REGARDING THE HIP JOINT:

1. The hip is a ball and socket joint. It is adapted to provide stability to your body at the expense of some freedom of movement. The hip joint has a capsule of unequal thickness and it is strengthened by ligaments. These ligaments together with the muscles limit the hip in its movements.

2. These muscles and the ligaments can be traumatized by a motion or motions that are exaggerated in any direction. Any lesion in your lumbar spine or your sacroiliac joint could cause one foot to "toe in" on one side and "toe out" on the other, and this may predispose you to a rotation lesion of one or both hip joints. Your gluteus muscles, the adduction, and the other hip-moving muscles may become tensed by a sacroiliac lesion. These are abnormal tensions, and may restrict movement of your hip.

3. You may complain of having difficulty in crossing your thighs while you are sitting or moving your thigh outward to reach your foot while getting dressed. Many symptoms of your hip will be referenced in your knee region. (See the

knee chapter.)

These are only suggested to give you an insight into what areas are involved in order to remain healthy and give you some idea what your physician has to master in order to provide you with the best care.

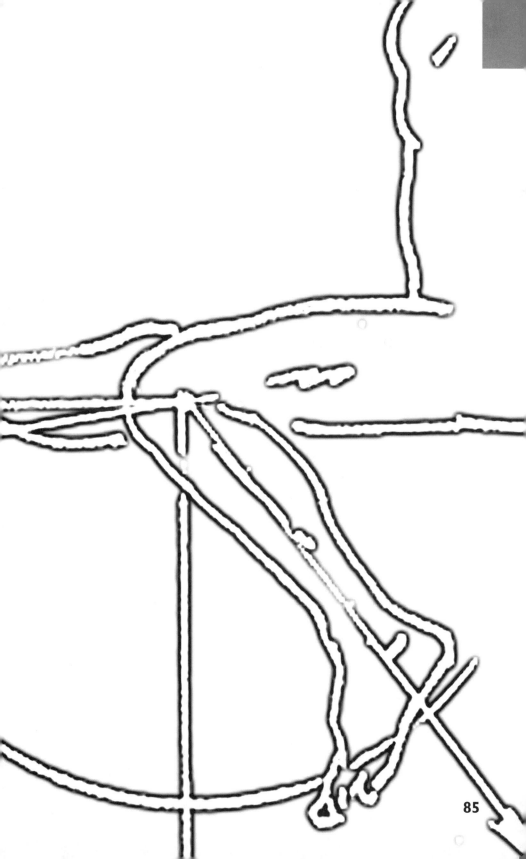

NOW TEST YOURSELF

(Please use a separate sheet of paper.)

1. With how many joints in your body do you walk?

2. What should you look for in the mirror?

3. Where does your back begin?

4. How do you develop bunions?

5. When does your posture become traumatized?

6. When should you compensate for leg length difference?

7. Are your bones rigid or plastic?

8. What condition stalks you?

9. At what age in children do bones ossify?

10. What are ligaments?

11. How can you create a lesion in your sacroiliac?

12. If you are stuck in a forward position should you move fast or slow? Why?

13. If you have trouble in any sacroiliac area, do you have a problem in another area? If so, where?

14. Nourishment to your sacroiliac joints comes from where?

15. Is the sacroiliac a fixed joint?

CHAPTER 8:

FEET AND LEGS

The feet of man
Have danced in joy
And marched to war
Have trampled in mud,
Upon the tiller's ground
Have followed solemnly
In mournful procession
Have jumped up and down
From counter and ladder
Walked in protest for some
Cause—Still they trod
Upon the highways of hope
'Til man learns to walk with his soul.

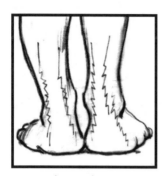

Valgus in Flat Feet
Pes Planus

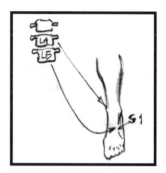

Nerve distribution

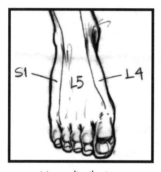

Nerve distribution

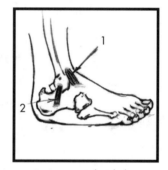

1. Anterior Talo Fibular
Ligament
2. Calcano Fibular Ligament

The distribution of some of the nerves to your feet

I t is important that you take good care of your feet at all times. You must become aware of how you walk, and how people around you walk. Do you walk evenly, or does your foot roll to one side? Does your shoe wear out more on your large toe side, or on the edge of your foot, or on the little-toe side?

You use every joint in your body to walk, including your jawbone. Be aware that chances are you bite hard when you are upset or during walking. When you experience a pain in your back or neck, or have a headache, think of your feet; then examine them. Why? Because most stresses in your body and most existing imbalances can be found in painful feet, or in a foot that doesn't cause you pain but is flat. It is likely that your feet may have been exposed to trauma some time in your past, even though you may not remember the incident. Your feet can shift the base plane of your spine and become a contributing cause of many problems in your body.

As your mind can hide problems, so can your body. This is called "masking." You may not be conscious of pain in your feet, but nevertheless, the feet may produce nerve irritations that your body must compensate for at a subconscious level. Do not neglect your feet, even to the point of making sure you prevent blisters or corns from forming.

You must wear a good pair of shoes, which should include a resilient cushion between your feet and the ground. Your shoe must have enough space to prevent pinching when your full body weight is on one foot, standing in one place, or when walking. Your shoe should distribute your weight in proper proportion. Make sure your shoe will at all times prevent your ankles from twisting. It should also have a flexible inner arch to permit your weight-bearing arch to function properly by allowing it to descend. Before you leave the store, look into the mirror to see that your lumbar spine maintains its normal curve of 1 1/2 inches. If it does not, the shoe is not right for you. Finally, your shoe must ventilate your feet properly. *(Do not tie your laces too tightly.)*

A patient of mine, Burt (not his real name), came to see me for a lower back problem resulting from lifting heavy objects as a foreman for a construction compa-

89

ny. During my examination, I asked that he remove the boots from his feet. He was not willing to do so at first. I asked him why he was reluctant to take off his boots. He said he was ashamed of how his feet looked and that he never removed his socks when he went to bed.

Now, I was more interested. I told him I wanted to see them for myself. Finally, he removed the socks and I saw his feet had the same greenish texture that I noticed on his hands. I asked him how this had happened. Burt told me that at some construction sites he picked up lumber, bricks and all kinds of objects that were infested with various fungi. He sought help from various dermatologists without any results, so he gave up and accepted the fact that this is the way he would have to live the rest of his life.

I told him there is a very simple solution to his problem and I would give it to him after I completed my examination and determined what kind of treatment he would need.

I asked him to buy a large bottle of castor oil and a large piece of soft flannel material, large enough to wrap his feet and legs. I told him to place them in a clean pair of socks to be used at night. For his hands he needed large gloves like potholders.

He was to warm the castor oil, removing the cap and placing the open bottle into hot water. Once warm, I told him to spread the oil on the flannel and wrap his both feet and both legs in it, and then place his feet in the socks during the night (so he wouldn't stain the sheets). He was to follow the same procedure on his hands and do this for one month. By that time I promised him he would see a great difference.

I asked him to use gloves to pick things up. After a week he noticed changes and after six weeks the fungi were gone. His back took longer to heal and when he was discharged I designed various exercises for him based on his x-rays. I believe that any and all exercises should be based upon the patient's individual x-rays.

This illustration shows the desired weight distribution on your foot.

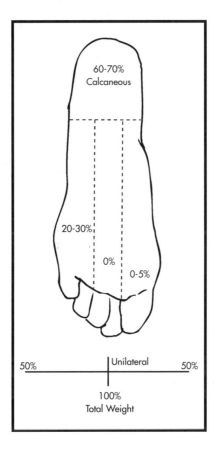

Static Weight Bearing

This next illustration shows the flow of your weight.

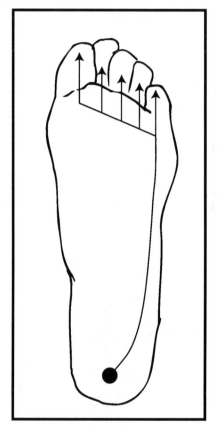

1. Feet must be directed straight forward.

2. 50% of total body weight on each foot.

3. Weight-bearing 60-70% must be on the calcaneus.

4. 20-20% of total body weight on outer weight-bearing arch and the fifth metatarsal.

5. 5-10% on the first metatarsal head.

6. 0% on the second and third metatarsal heads.

Flow of Weight

THINGS TO REMEMBER

Your back begins at the soles of your feet, and it is never too late to begin to take care of your feet. Regardless of your age, everybody needs to maintain good foot care. Additional points to ensure healthy feet include:

1. Maintain 50 percent of your body weight on each foot in order to maintain the weight-bearing arch. This is a must to remember: Shifting all your weight on one foot will hurt your back sooner or later and will cause other problems.

2. Maintain good muscle tone to prevent your arches from falling.

3. *(This is for ladies and gentlemen alike.)* Keep the heel height at a minimum to prevent your body weight from shifting forward into the shoe; otherwise, the arch cannot be maintained. Your feet will end up jammed into the toe of the shoe regardless of the length of the shoe.

4. Keep the weight off of your second and third toes to prevent a condition known as metatarsalgia, which will create pain and discomfort in your feet.

5. If more than 10% of your body weight is on your big toe, you are bound to develop bunions.

6. If the heel of your shoe is more than 1 1/2 inches thicker than the sole, then the lumbar curve will be larger than 1 1/2 inches; this will cause low back pain. A 2 inch lumbar curve is always pathological. Become conscious of this fact so you will not suffer low back pain, especially as a result of high heels.

7. If your heel height is low, and your lumbar curve is less than 1 inch, you will also have low back pain. This is also pathological.

8. Your shoes have the ability to maintain good foot and body relations, or they can destroy the mechanical requirements for the proper erect position of your body.

The following illustration shows how to adjust your toes by traction, or joint separation. This should be done rhythmically with a gentle movement. This will break up soft tissue that has hardened, and will return good range of movement and aid in proper circulation.

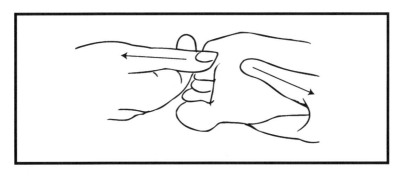

Manipulation of the phalanges is principally traction or joint separation. Such manipulation, intermittent and rhythmical, breaks fibrous restriction to motion and facilitates the return of circulation.

This next illustration shows how to reduce a bunion by straightening the toe. Be gentle; it would be best if a professional does this.

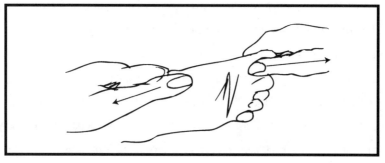

Hallux (the big toe) should be straightened by traction

This next illustration shows how to care for your feet. Hold the foot gently; do not use pressure. Use gentle massage. Do not try to find pressure points. Your feet are very delicate; you do not want to bruise the covering of the bones.

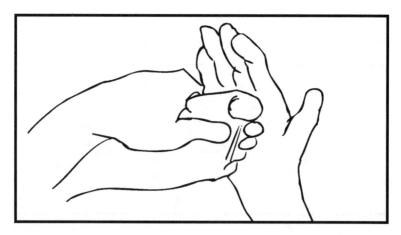

The following illustration shows how all foot corrections are made. This position is essential in restoring normalcy to the metatarsal bones.

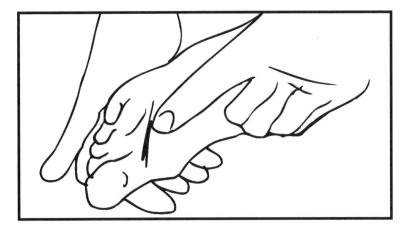

The metatarsal or distal end of the longitudinal arch is cupped in the palm and the arch elevated. This restores normal position and the shaft of the metatarsal bones may be grasped without trauma to the interosseous tissues. This is an essential position of all foot correction except in pes-cavus, abnormally high longitudinal arch.

This next illustration shows how to increase the range of motion in the direction flexion.

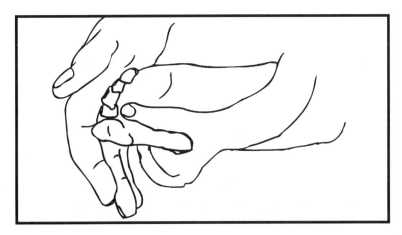

Increasing the range of motion is necessary in the direction of plantar flexion at the metatarso-phalangial (foot and toes) articulation for hallux flexus to hallux rigidus.

This next illustration shows how each toe should be put through its complete range of motion.

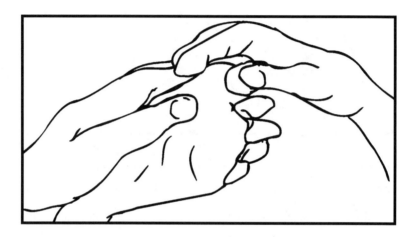

LEGS

Legs are usually of unequal length. In my practice I have found this condition to be functional, not anatomical, in nature. Over 80% of all my patients showed actual leg length differences. Of these, about 50% of the functional shortness was on one side. The common difference is less than 1 centimeter. This small difference in the leg contributes to problems in the sacroiliac area, but it also indicates a problem in the upper neck area, mainly on the short leg. A compensation shows on the same side in the upper neck as well.

If your legs have a difference of more than one centimeter, then the walking error is greater and your posture will in time be affected. As this is not a true anatomical shortness, it must have come into existence due to internal muscle spasms of your

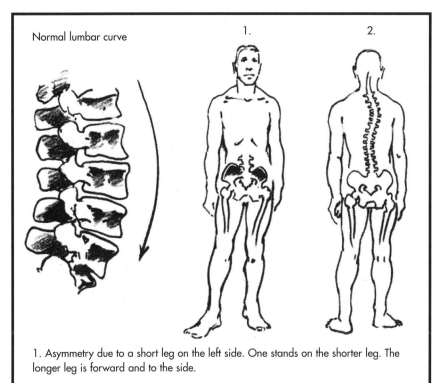

1. Asymmetry due to a short leg on the left side. One stands on the shorter leg. The longer leg is forward and to the side.

2. Functional curvature or scoliosis. Tilted shoulder (right). Feet nearly together.

back, called psoasitis, on the short side. When your lumbar muscles are unequal, they become tense and your hip may be in spasm. The ligaments in the back of your feet may become lengthened or shortened, and your legs appear to be of unequal length, when in actuality they are not. Of course, your leg may become shorter or longer if it is fractured. Shortness can also be caused by infection, and growth can be arrested due to trauma, polio, or neuritis.

Congenital leg length differences can be as much as 4 full inches. In that case, the head of the femur and the greater trochanter were malformed. When I was visiting Israel with my wife, I was asked to help a young woman who had such a deformity. Her hips had been malformed since infancy. I was able to break up the hardened

97

adhesions and helped to restore circulation into the area. She was then able to walk with greater ease. Years later this woman had reconstructive surgery and today she lives a normal life.

If you have more than one centimeter of difference in your legs, compensation will result. Regardless of how small the difference, the chances are that you may develop some functional disturbance in your sacroiliac area. If you develop such a disturbance, remember that these are easily corrected. However, when your sacroiliac area or pelvis becomes injured, and when one leg is shorter than one centimeter, then the problem becomes more pronounced. Never forget that your bones are quite plastic and they will become deformed under stress of any kind, regardless of your age. I have seen this in gardeners, masons, office workers, people who sit all day at the computer. I have seen this in people in all walks of life from all occupations. Stress is the shadow that stalks us all. You cannot eliminate it entirely, but you can reduce its influence.

If you have a chronic sacroiliac or pelvic condition, this has been built up ever since you began to walk. (I am assuming that you have not had an accident that precipitated this condition.) A chronic sacroiliac with a twisted back does not always cause pain, and you may not need any treatment to correct it. You may be able to function quite well. However, if you develop pain, you must seek professional help. You do not have to get used to the pain. There is no need to suffer.

Now I want you to understand the intelligence your body uses in order to help you. In order for your body to perform the tasks you demand of it, it shifts your weight disproportionately toward the long leg side. This does not mean that your long leg is the normal one and the short leg is abnormal. Both are normal, but the long leg carries the weight and strikes the ground harder, with the result that your ilium rocks backward, causing your sacrum to become flexed and lowered on that side. This causes the tilt of your sacrum to be diminished. On the other side, the ilium is pulled forward on the short leg side, causing that side of the sacrum to go backward and elevating the top of your sacrum at the same time.

Your doctor will correct this condition, known as compensatory sacral correction toward the short leg side. When this is done, no scoliosis of a functional nature can develop.

If your sacral top is not level, or both ends are not level, compensation usually results in your back developing a scoliosis. In 70-75% of all scoliosis cases, the condition can be improved quite satisfactorily if you are under 50 years of age, and helped considerably even if you are over 50.

Become aware of your body. Every hour of the day, stop what you are doing and focus your attention on the muscles in your hands, arms, legs, and feet. Focus on how your feet feel under your weight. Are they comfortable? If not, why? Now ask yourself: Are my legs and hips tight because of my feet?

Next, bring your attention to the muscles of your back. Feel their tightness. Now, relax them by taking a deep breath, and clasp your hands in front of your chest. While you hold your arms and hands six inches away from your body, press your hands together as hard as you can. Then, exhale and release them. This will relax the muscles of your back between the shoulders.

Come back to your feet and legs. Learn to relax them while you are sitting: elevate them and extend your knees, one leg at a time. When you sit for prolonged periods of time, you place pressure on the circulatory system in your legs. You must consciously contract the muscles of your legs as these muscles actively cause the flow of blood against gravity up into your heart. Prolonged sitting is not healthy. If you must sit for long periods, elevate your legs. If your job requires you to stand all day long, walk up and down several times, every hour, as much as possible.

When you are not working, keep your feet up to aid blood circulation, especially if you have varicose veins. Any leg exercises you do that require your feet to be above your head will be beneficial for everyone.

Once you have learned to know your body, you will have learned how to avert serious problems before they become acute and damage your health. Come to know your own weaknesses. Get rid of your pressures. Each pressure is a trigger point

....

that can cause the deterioration of your health. Prevent these from taking root in your body, in your mind, in your emotions. Learn each day to know your life and your spirit.

HELP OR TREATMENT

If after diagnosis, treatment is required for the short leg, be sure that the pelvis is also treated. An imbalance in the pelvis will contribute to the illusion of anatomically short leg. In children, you must watch to be sure that the bones develop properly. The bones do not complete their ossification (closure) before the child reaches his/her 17th or 18th birthday.

When my children were young, I always stretched the heel of each foot so that they would carry their weight equally on each foot. The heel carries most of the weight of the body. Make sure your children's feet are taken care of. Do not wait to treat feet problems when the feet are fully grown. Gentle massage is helpful, especially before the child is put to bed.

A good doctor must also be a good engineer in order to design the best method of treatment for you. If your leg is longer on the left, the vertebrae in your low back will rotate to the right. And if your leg is longer on the right, the vertebrae in your low back will rotate to the left. In this case, even if your lumbar is rotated to the high side, no heel change is needed. The doctor will increase the forward/backward lumbar curve and the vertebrae will release and begin to move to the low side.

Remember that too much heel correction can cause damage. It is better to lower the longer leg instead of raising the shorter one. Before accepting treatment of any kind on your back as a result of shortness in one leg, make sure that the primary cause is removed; otherwise, you will have recurring problems.

If you have unequal leg lengths and this does not bother you, don't correct it. But my patients with leg-length discrepancy that did have symptoms of low back pain or pain in the upper neck became symptom-free after corrections. They did not need heel lifts of any kind. In all the decades of my practice, I never gave or recommended a heel change, except in anatomically short legs or through fracture when corrective shoes were necessary.

Now, let's discuss your ligaments. These are bands of connective tissue holding all your bones together. Do not expect your ligaments in your back, hands, feet, or knees to have the same characteristics as another person's. They are different in everyone. You may have heavy, rigid ligaments; or you may have lighter, rigid ligaments. Or your ligaments may be heavy elastic or light elastic. The combinations are numerous. Therefore, treatment for your problems will be different than the next person's. Mobility testing by itself is useless, because what you consider normal mobility in your low back will be abnormal for someone else.

The sacroiliac joint, which supports your lumbar and all other vertebrae, including your head, depends entirely upon the ligaments for its stability. These ligaments are so strong that it would take enormous force to cause them to rupture. Yet a small amount of force, such as a wrong move or a sudden twist, may affect them. The discs in your back and the sacroiliac joint suffer more wear and tear than any other part in your body. These undergo constant strain while trying to adjust to the daily load placed on them. Consider that with all the abuse your back and this joint receives during your lifetime how well they hold up! Even so, they are vulnerable to occasional breakdowns.

How many ways can you injure your sacroiliac? Consider only one for the present: driving a car. You can injure this area by simply slamming hard on the brakes. Your ilium can move on your sacrum and the end result is a strain, and, at worst, the pubic bone may move and become subluxated. Your ilium and your pubic bone are one complete whole. If your ilium moves backward toward the seat of your car, your pubic bone on the same side will move up. If your ilium moves forward, the pubic bone will move down. However, sooner or later the opposite ilium will move to compensate to lessen the damage.

If you should be "stuck" in a forward bent position, do not attempt to move quickly. Your sacroiliac joint may have fluid shifting toward the backside. You should wait; give it a little time to normalize. Then, moving slowly, very slowly, stand up. By the time you are in the erect position, the fluid will be nearly even in the front and the back compartments of your sacroiliac joint.

Never make fast movements of any kind with your back. If you play tennis or if you are a golfer, your injuries will occur more frequently in the sacroiliac area and low lumbar region. I had to teach many golfers how to stand so that they would prevent injuries. Besides damaging the sacroiliac joints, the knee can also be damaged, which then causes stress on the hips. Every golfer should look in the mirror to see which shoulder is higher and position the leg on that side at least one inch behind the other. That way, compensation will take place prior to play and not after an injury. The weight of the body must always be on the heel and must turn with the swing so that the knee does not become strained.

You should remember that if you have trouble in one sacroiliac area, there is always a secondary problem in the other sacroiliac area or joint as well as in the lower lumbar vertebrae. If and when you need help, remember to treat both joints, not just the one that hurts, or else your problem will recur. A quick fix is not the answer.

Nourishment to your sacroiliac joints comes from the fifth lumbar and the first and second sacral nerves. Do not ignore the lower lumbar vertebrae in maintaining good health. When a problem arises in the lumbar vertebrae, the pain is often felt in the sacroiliac joints. You will believe that it is the joints of your sacroiliac producing the pain, but quite often the sacroiliac joints will reflect pain into the lumbar area, and you will mistake this as having a lumbar origin. Therefore, a good diagnosis is important to identify the primary lesion. To help your doctor, always indicate exactly where the pain is located. Do this with your fingers. If you use your whole hand, you are telling your doctor that the pain generalized, which means it can come from your lumbar or sacroiliac regions.

If your pain is acute and comes on suddenly, and if you are a woman, it may be from your uterus, bladder, or rectum. If you are a man, it may be from your prostate, bladder, or rectum. Also note that should your pain increase after you go to bed but lessen when you get up and move around, it most likely is from your sacroiliac area. If the pain grows worse as the day progresses and you find relief by lying down, it is most likely of lumbar origin or involves a disc.

The reason there are so many problems in this area is that the sacrum or sacroiliac joint is not a fixed joint. It moves and glides constantly, slipping from one bone to another. Therefore, you must not put all your weight on one side or the other for any length of time; you will stretch the ligaments and, in time, injure yourself.

Face your fears
Run not from them
You alone gave birth to them
You alone can dissolve them.

CHAPTER 9 EXAMINATION

NOW TEST YOURSELF

(Please use a separate sheet of paper.)

1. Is rest always the best treatment? Under what conditions?

2. Which muscle is responsible for a bent back?

3. Which muscle flexes your thigh in a reclining position?

4. Why are discs "rigid"?

5. How is nutrition taken in by discs?

6. What part of the cartilage plate contains the growth zone?

7. What is muscular rheumatism?

8. Does fibrous tissue shorten or lengthen?

9. How can rigidity in connective tissue be overcome?

10. What should you consider when you experience lumbago?

11. Can depression or a common cold interfere with nutrition to a joint?

12. What is arthritis?

13. Should you ignore a cramp in your back?

14. What conditions can bad posture cause?

15. Can anger cause pain in your back?

16. Why is your shoulder susceptible to strain or trauma?

CHAPTER 9:

LUMBAR REGION

Move through your pains
Do not dwell in them.
Do not hold onto them
Release them and you will
begin to heal.

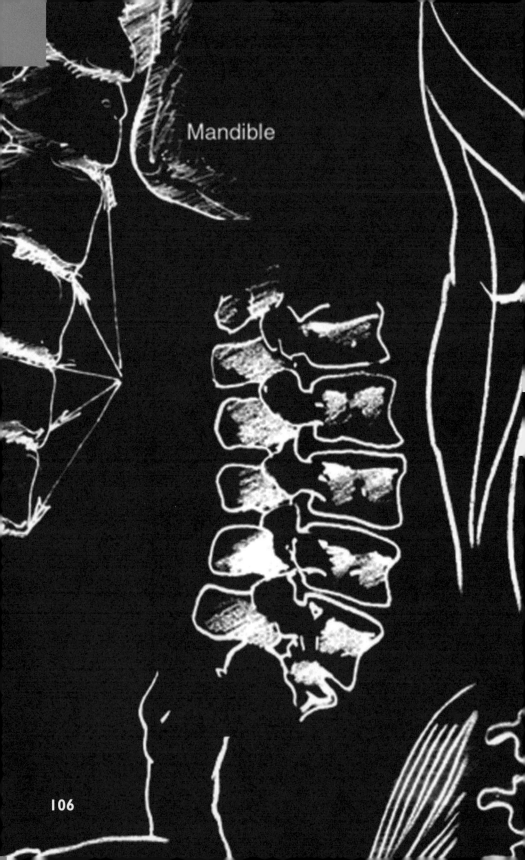

Mandible

O ver the years you have heard your friends complain or maybe even you have complained of low back pain under various names. The most commonly used name is lumbago; the second most common name is sciatica. I am here to set the record straight: Lumbago is not sciatic pain; sciatic pain is nerve-related.

What Is Lumbago?

Any discomfort in the lumbar area of your back is lumbago.

What Causes Lumbago?

1. Unequal leg length
2. Lesions of the sacroiliac joint
3. The base plane of the sacroiliac joint is unbalanced

These three are the most common causes of lumbago. Other causes include:

4. Inflammation of your psoas muscles
5. Disc injury
6. Spondylolisthesis (the forward displacement of a vertebra over a lower segment, usually of the fourth or fifth lumbar vertebra)
7. Myofibrositis (inflammation of muscle fibrils; especially muscle covering sheaths). (Myofibril is a slender thread of muscle fiber composed of filaments.)
8. Tumors of the spinal cord or the brain
9. Arthritis
10. Fractures
11. Abnormalities of the feet or of one foot
12. Problems caused under anesthesia, such as subluxation or adjustment while sedated
13. Posture (consider your occupation; curvatures of the spine can be due to stress)
14. Pain caused by reflex from another area
15. A cold settling in the back ("chilled to the bone")

16. Emotional trauma

17. Mental attitude, such as hysteria

18. Combinations of the above, plus other factors not enumerated here

Your doctor will examine your spine by checking your legs and feet as well as lesions in the sacroiliac to see if your base is off balance. He or she will then check for muscle pathology, which you experience as acute strain that could be complicated by some form of infection or a cold.

Whether you or your doctor recommends rest, remember that rest is a wonderful way to start healing. However, often rest can mask a poor method of treatment.

Many physicians overlook lower back pain originating at least partially from the psoas muscles. If you should have a bent back or your spine becomes distorted, the muscle responsible is the psoas. Your doctor may well decide that the cause is your lower thoracic and upper lumbars, forgetting that the main nerve supply comes to the psoas muscle from this area.

When you are in a reclining position, the function of the psoas muscle is to flex the thigh on the groin. When you stand upright, the two muscles on each side stabilize your lumbar spine. The psoas muscles are sensitive to strain and infections, such as infections of the mouth and teeth, prostatitis, the common cold, or venereal disease through blood circulation. Inflammation of the psoas muscles on both sides is rare. A typical lumbar scoliosis is one that is held fixed by a one-sided fibrotic psoas.

Every day, breathe yourself into your body and know you are alive. Realize that whatever weakens you, weakens your body; whatever strengthens you, strengthens your body.

INTERVERTEBRAL DISC

Your disc is one of the nine ligaments holding your spine together. Their pathology (or, disease, is a change in the tissue, which cause or are caused by disease) can be divided into chronic and acute. One is caused by the wear and tear of normal activity, and one is caused by a sudden injury, including severe strain.

Young persons will often exhibit disc changes in their spine on their x-rays. Many discs are rigid. Their nutrient channels are injured, and the result is that the joint or segments of the vertebrae become desiccated and immobile, yielding a stiff back. If you experience an unbalanced pelvis, attend to it immediately, as this is probably the single most predisposing cause of injury to the disc and lumbar problems. You do not ever need to suffer with this condition.

Mobility is an absolute necessity to keep the discs in your spine healthy. The nutrition your disc receives is through the minute perforations in the cartilage plate. As your spine moves, the nutrient fluid is taken into the disc and forced out. Anything that limits motion in your spine, especially after you are 80, tends to reduce the fluidity of the disc and render it rigid. When your discs become rigid, normalcy can never be returned, but their function can be improved by breaking down the fibrous tissue that causes ankylosis, a consolidation of the joint from disease, injury, or a surgical procedure.

Remember that all lesions in your spine are always accompanied by some form of subluxation, which is itself an injury requiring treatment.

The cartilage plate, which is a part of the body of the vertebra, has a dual purpose. The surface, which is contiguous to the body of the vertebra, contains its growth zone. This is a most important part of your vertebra. The other side aids in enclosing and protecting the disc, and serves as an anchor for the attachment of many fibers, an elongated thread-like structure.

Muscular rheumatism is nothing other than myofibrositis or fibrositis. Muscular rheumatism can be the cause of a large majority of lumbagos, both acute and chronic. Acute refers to muscular elements; chronic is more of a fibrositis (inflammation of the filaments, the fine slender threads of muscle fiber). Many factors are involved, including an unbalanced pelvis, vertebral lesions, strain, bad posture, fatigue, constipation, urates (carbonic acid salt found in urine), bad tonsils, sinus infection, gonorrhea, hemorrhoids, prostatitis, diseases of the uterus, kidney pathology, or nervousness. All of these are conditions for which you need medical treatment.

Fibrous tissue that produces muscular rheumatism is like a vine that strangles. It entwines itself until it chokes the structure to death. Fibrous tissue thickens and short- ens. If when you wake up one morning and feel stiff—just a little—and you bend down to pick up your shoe and you feel and hear a snap and then cannot move or you fall down, then your back will hurt each time you try to move. What you have is a fibrositic condition that has been ignored over the years.

An acute lumbago, on the other hand, can be forcibly re-adjusted to relieve the nerve irritation in the joint by stretching the fibrotic tissue so that the condition should not recur.

Many strains occur, and when they hurt a little, you place very little importance on them. However, these are capable of deforming or choking the structure they are attached to. These are fascia (fibrous tissue around a muscle and various organs) strains. These fasciae are often overlooked in examination, and their importance is ignored. But they are of prime importance. You should never be treated for the effect of the pain instead of the cause.

Rigidity of connective tissue can be overcome by stretching it beyond its elastic limit so that the shortened fibers give up their chokehold. Lumbar and sacroiliac sub- luxations often take place while you are undergoing surgery, while you are under deep anesthesia, or when you are being removed from the operating table or after delivery of a child. These are marked by acute pain. A firm pillow should always be placed under the lumbar spine to avoid accidents in the operating room. This is rarely done, as it is not considered important enough.

When you experience the pain of lumbago, consider first the condition of your feet. Any stress or imbalance in your feet will contribute to lumbago. Even painless flat feet may tilt the sacral base and subconsciously cause mechanical or nervous reflex- es that will affect the lumbar and the upper spine as well. (See the chapter on feet.)

WHAT IS ARTHRITIS?

Illness may be a disordered human spirit
Needing re-organization
Before healing can set in.

Arthritis is an inflammation of a joint marked by pain, heat, redness, and swelling. There are many different inflammatory conditions, and many different names for each of them. Some are due to gout, some are chronic (for example, rheumatoid). Some are due to psoriasis. Some are osteo- (bone) arthritis. Children have their own arthritic conditions. Some are from tuberculosis, but most are from nutritional diseases, such as faulty calcium metabolism, which is governed by the parathyroid and the liver. You may, of course, be predisposed to arthritis by your genetic inheritance.

Infections such as streptococcus and venereal diseases can interfere with nutrition to the joints. Conditions such as depression and the common cold also increase the inflammation of a joint or joints. There are many more contributing causes for arthritis, and it is good to be informed about the various causes to prevent this condition.

If you experience a painful inflammation in your spine, you can obtain relief by relaxing the muscles in your spine and stretching the ligaments that surround them. I said earlier that when the vertebrae are out of balance, nutrition is impeded to that area. This imbalance puts stress on the entire spine. When this stress is relieved then nutrition is restored to the affected area.

Your spine is as vulnerable to fractures as any other bone in your body. Your spine transmits all the nerves to every part of your body. Injury to the spinal cord can create problems from a simple limp to paralysis. Respect your spine and you will enjoy your health.

Any minor accident may in time produce severe symptoms. Never overlook a fractured rib. If you experience a cramp in your back, don't ignore it; it may be a fractured rib. Be careful and watch your posture. If you sit, do not slouch. You have but one body to last you a lifetime. The quality of this life depends largely on the care you give yourself. Bad posture due to laziness or carelessness can predispose you to pain and disease and can cause your internal organs to prolapse—to be squashed.

Be aware that you may develop a curvature of your spine by constant sitting and watching TV or by reading for hours. Don't be sedentary. Change your habits! This is the recommended treatment, but much of it depends on your willingness to change.

Many pains are thought to originate in the lower back, but these actually may come from the feet, abdomen, pelvis, internal organs, and infections, or even from an argument with someone. Anger has a way of giving pain, in the low back as well as the upper back and neck area. Remember that anger removes knowledge, and knowledge is the light everyone needs.

Always create the time to keep your body and its joints in motion. When you move, you prove to yourself that you live. When your joints move, they will help you prolong and maintain good health.

X-rays cannot reveal the extent of your pain; they are shadows on shadows. Your x-rays may be normal when examined but pain may persist. Arthritic pain, for example, is seldom found on x-rays, although arthritic changes are. Do not get discouraged. Prevent arthritic pain by following these simple steps:

1. Keep moving. Do not live a sedentary existence.

2. Take care of your spine. Doing so will help to improve nerve and blood supply to all joints and internal organs.

3. Eat well and play well.

4. Have your back examined at least once a year by a competent chiropractor, osteopath, or doctor who knows how to relieve spine pressures.

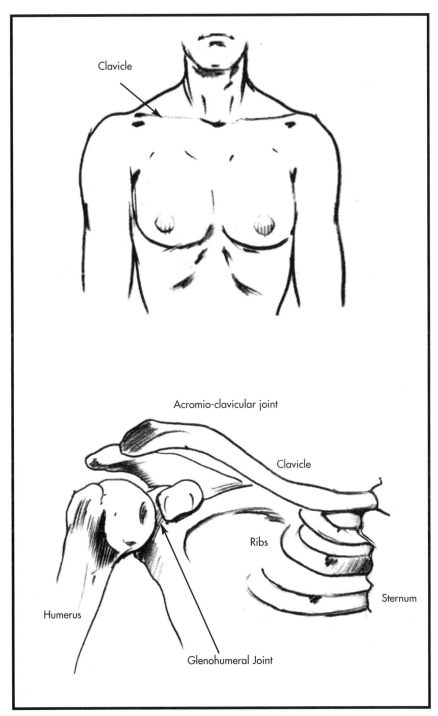

Anatomy Of The Shoulder

. . . .

YOUR SHOULDER GIRDLE

Your upper limbs are attached to your body by three bones: the humerus (upper arm), the scapula (shoulder blade), and the clavicle (collarbone). The upper arm is a long, thin bone and is the largest bone of your upper body. It has a hemispherical head that fits into a cavity of the scapula called the glenoid cavity. Your shoulder blade is a flat, triangular bone that forms the back part of your shoulder girdle. Your collarbone is a slender, curved bone that lies horizontally at the root of the neck in the upper part of your chest. These are all interdependent, not just functionally but structurally.

For movement to occur in your upper body, it must start in the glenoid cavity by the long bone or upper arm, which is supplemented by the scapular and motion of the clavicle at the sternum and a mutual action of the clavicle at the acromioclavicular joint. If movement is impaired at one point, it will require increased movement elsewhere, which will overtax one of the other joints, causing a secondary lesion, with the result that symptoms will arise at a distance from their root cause. Never be fooled by symptoms, and never treat symptoms alone.

For example, if you develop a sacroiliac lesion, this could easily limit the mobility in the glenohumeral joint (where the head of your arm joins the glenoid cavity) by producing tension on the long muscle of your lower back (the latissimus dorsi muscle). When your collarbone is restricted in its movement, your shoulder blade becomes susceptible to a lesion in its relation to the collarbone because the unhampered shoulder blade may move beyond the limit of the range of the collarbone.

Therefore, whenever there is a lesion between the shoulder blade and the collarbone, the collarbone fibers of your trapezius muscles and your deltoid muscle will not act in harmony with the scapular fibers of the same two muscles. This condition is often wrongly diagnosed as subdeltoid bursitis.

Your shoulder joint is similar to the hip joint. Because of the great range of movement of your shoulder joint, simple synovitis becomes infrequent. Thus, whenever you experience pain and/or muscle spasms, and these prevent your joints from moving, you should always consider the possibility of a serious problem—such as a disease of the joint—especially when there is no trauma to the shoulder. Because the glenoid cavity is shallow, it makes the shoulder susceptible to strain and to trauma.

The muscles of your shoulder must always be relaxed. If you have pain, do not move your arm and shoulder beyond the point of your pain.

A dropped shoulder is usually due to a trauma where your clavicle becomes more prominent than the bone on the opposite side. Your shoulder has freedom of movement, and its stability is sacrificed to remain free. The muscles that surround your shoulder girdle limit the movement of your shoulder.

1. Your shoulder may be susceptible to the production of lesions from your spine by cutting off the nerve supply.

2. Also, the nerve supply will be cut off by a short leg or a sacroiliac lesion on the same side by increasing tension on the latissimus dorsi muscle.

3. If you make exaggerated movements, occupational in nature, due to sports activity, a fall, fatigue or even by the arms just hanging lazily by your side, the nerve supply from your neck and upper back will be strained.

The symptoms of shoulder joint lesion, primary or secondary, are:
1. Restricted movement at the joint
2. Pain, increased by certain movements

TREATMENT OF THE SHOULDER JOINT
In the treatment, you must consider all of these:
1. Muscles related to the joint
2. Lesions of the spine
3. Ribs or the pelvis
These could exert an abnormal influence upon the shoulder or shoulder girdle.
4. Any lesion found anywhere in the shoulder girdle must be removed or reduced.
5. Soft tissue muscle treatment should be carried out only on those shoulder

muscles found to have abnormal tissue quality.

6. Look for swollen (edematous) or fibrotic muscle. However, if there is hemorrhage into the muscle, no manipulation or massage of any kind should be done.

7. When you cannot turn your arm inward, the tension is usually found in the teres minor muscle and the inferior spinatus.

8. When your arm cannot rotate outward, it may be caused by spasm of the sub scapularis, the latissimus dorsi, the pectoralis, or fibers from the deltoid or inflammation of the capsule or the subdeltoid bursa.

9. Never allow anyone to manipulate your shoulder by force against painful muscle spasms.

SHOULDER: RANGE OF MOTION

These are the normal degrees of rotation. Test yourself gently.

Abduction	180°
Adduction	45°
Flexion	90°
Extension	45°
Internal Rotation	55°
External Rotation	40-45°

ROTATOR CUFF

You probably have heard much about the rotator cuff. Degeneration and tearing of its tendon of insertion restricts the movement of the shoulder, especially in abduction. The cuff is composed of four muscles: the supraspinatus (abducts your arm), infraspinatus (rotates your arm sideways), teres minor (SIT) muscle (rotates the arm sideways), and the subscapularis (rotates the arm medially). This area is injured most frequently by a fall or careless exercise.

Your shoulders have a range of motion like no other part of the body, and allows you to perform a myriad of activity. For this reason, your shoulders are more likely to suffer injuries. The most common ones are dislocation, sprain, separation and fractures.

Dislocation: When your arm is jerked backward or pulled sharply, the head of the upper arm may come out of your shoulder socket. Numbness, swelling and bruising may occur.

Sprain and separation: These are caused by a fall on your shoulder. A sprain results when your ligaments are torn. The sprain might be a small tear or large enough that the acromion (top of the shoulder) and your clavicle (collarbone) separate.

Fracture: This happens during a heavy fall on your shoulder. The fracture is usually on the neck of the humerus (upper arm) often caused by a fall on an outstretched arm or elbow.

There is also an ailment called the frozen shoulder when the shoulder joint is stiff and restricted in motion.

It is important to follow the exercise program your doctor recommends.

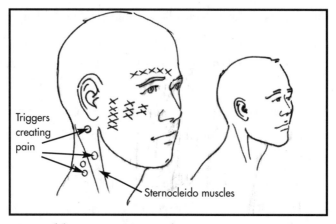

Triggers creating pain

Sternocleido muscles

Use cold water or ice cubes on your muscles in the front and back of your neck. Pain will diminish with each application.

THE STERNOCLEIDO MUSCLE

A neck muscle, the sternocleido, is one of the most prominent muscles of the shoulder girdle. It is important for three reasons:

1. It frequently is the site of hematomas (blood clots) that may cause the neck to turn to one side (wry neck). A blood clot in this area—or any other area in the body—should not be ignored, especially after an injury.

2. The lymph nodes become enlarged as a result of infection.

3. It is traumatized in hyperextension injuries of the neck, such as whiplash.

In auto accidents especially this muscle injury is often overlooked. It is frequently an undiagnosed component of a whiplash injury. Note also that it occurs as a result of falls, particularly in skiing accidents.

Do not turn your back
On the outside world, and look toward
The inner world only,
Look toward the world as it is—

Look toward another
Human being—look to God—
Toward life! Begin to live!

CHAPTER 10 EXAMINATION

NOW TEST YOURSELF

(Please use a separate sheet of paper.)

1. What kind of joint is your knee?

2. What are the most obvious movements of your knee?

3. When does a lesion most likely occur in your knee?

4. What are predisposing lesions of your knee?

5. If your knees become swollen, what should you do?

CHAPTER 10:

YOUR KNEE JOINT

Bow not your head

nor

Flex your knees

to Failures past

Pay

no homage to hatred,

anger

or your fears

Find

your strength to release

all these!

Balance

your human spirit now!

For

in this very moment

you

your judgment in your hand

hold.

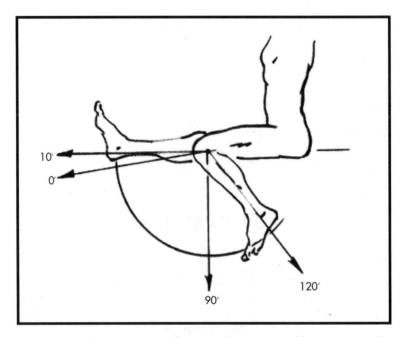

Range of motion of your knee in flexion and extension

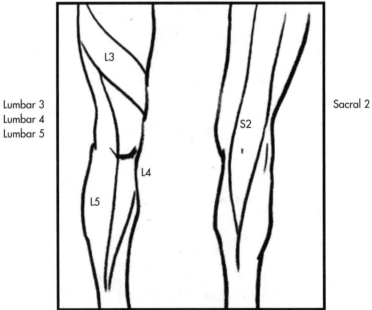

Nerves to the knee

Your knee is a hinge joint that does not fit together well, so it must depend upon ligaments and muscles for stability. The most obvious movement of your knee is flexion-extension. Your knee moves forward in extension and backward in flexion. Your femur rotates medially as the joint locks in extreme extension. The other active motion of the joint is rotation by the individual action of the hamstrings when your knee is flexed to a right angle. The biceps femoris muscles (extends the thigh; flexes and rotates your leg sideways) produce an outward rotation of your leg and the combined action of the semitendinous (flexes and rotates your leg medially; also extends the thigh) and semimembranous (flexes the leg and extends the thigh) produce inward rotation. Minor or passive movements are permitted at your knee when all the muscles are relaxed. These slight movements are abduction, adduction, rotation, and gliding medially (toward the other knee) and laterally (outward). These movements may be limited by a lesioned knee. Abduction separates the surfaces on the medial side and places tension on the medial collateral ligament; adduction does the opposite. When there is rotation, it involves the femur or the tibia. If there is an internal rotation of your femur at your knee, it is the same as an external rotation of your tibia.

A lesion in your knee occurs when the minor protective movements are exaggerated to a point producing trauma. This may happen through violent contact with an object or by rotation against resistance at your joint, such as locking your knee and turning beyond the limit of your knee's natural resistance. Lesions produced during abduction are by an external force applied medially to the lateral side of your knee. A lesion produced in adduction is by a force to the medial side of the knee and directed laterally while the ankle and hip are in a relative fixed position.

Your subjective symptoms will be:

1. localized pain
2. decreased range of movement
3. freedom of voluntary movements
4. painful locking in a semifixed position, indicating that the medial meniscus (a

cres cent-shaped cartilage in the knee joint) may be displaced and immobilized
between the surfaces of the joint. This is not a lesion by itself; nevertheless, it
complicates the picture.

5. no inflammatory swelling occurs in an uncomplicated lesion of your knee

6. if there is inflammatory swelling, it will be a crescent-shaped fullness near
your patella (kneecap). This may indicate a lesion of a serious nature with a
possible displacement or damage to the medial meniscus, especially if the knee
becomes locked in partial flexion.

Predisposing lesions of your knee are the following:

1. pes planus—flat foot or feet

2. eversion of the foot (turning out of the foot)
*These two combined will require accommodation at the knee in walking,
causing the knee to become predisposed to rotation or abduction lesioning.*

3. Internal or external rotation lesion of the hip joint will predispose the knee to a
rotation lesion.

4. A sacroiliac lesion by its alteration in tension on muscles and fascia affect the
knee near its extremes of movement.

5. A primary lesion of the second lumbar vertebra may predispose the knee through
the nerve supply from that vertebra.

6. Rotation lesion in the lower lumbar may be a cause on a mechanical base (i.e.,
it is not a disease). Also, a "toeing in" of one foot and "toeing out" of the other
foot is not organic (not a disease) but is also a mechanical base.

7. If your knee becomes swollen and painful to treat, use a 2" bandage of thin, pure
rubber starting well below the knee. Wrap it comfortably around the knee. Do
not leave it on longer than 5 minutes. The bandage produces some anesthesia
because of its pressure, which induces relaxation and helps to reduce the
swelling. The bandage should be loosened and reapplied. See your physician as
soon as possible.

You likely do not think much about your knees on a daily basis unless you are in pain or if you wear a skirt or dress above them. Your knees are susceptible to injury from normal wear and tear, from participation in sports, fitness activity, and from your daily household chores.

Both women and men are subject to knee pain, such as torn cartilage, tendonitis, fracture, sprains and tears of the cruciate ligament ACL (anterior cruciate ligament). The risk is greater with sports that involve jumping, pivoting or quick de-celerations, such as basketball, soccer, and skiing. Even a wrong move in an aerobic class can tear the ACL. You will hear a "pop" as your knee gives way.

You may have painful kneecaps, such as bursitis (protective sac inflamed), tendinitis (tendons attach to knee cap, chondromalacia), or runners knee (protective cartilage is worn out). Rest is the treatment, as well as modification of activity. Surgery should be a last resort.

To prevent knee injury:

1. Warm up before working out.
2. Avoid sudden increase in activity or duration of activity.
3. Strengthen front and back leg muscles.
4. Wear appropriate athletic shoes.

Sprains and strains—Knee injury can be treated by applying RICE. RICE = Rest, Ice, Compression and Elevation.

Tendonitis is more serious. It involves inflammation of a tendon, with swelling, redness, and pain. Vigorous exercises will bring on tendonitis. When tendons or ligaments are torn, they require surgery. Twisting your knee can cause bursitis and bring on inflammation with some pain. When pain lasts for more than 72 hours, or makes it impossible to walk, and you hear popping from your knees, see your doctor and have them evaluated to prevent life-long problems. Exercise regularly to avoid arthritis. Control your weight. (Being overweight is an important cause of arthritis in the knees.) Don't over-exercise. When pain is present, see your doctor.

Relief for arthritis

1. Warm bath or shower—never hot
2. Mild stretching exercises. This will loosen the knee joint.
3. Capsicum cream. It's made from hot peppers and when applied to the knee will generate heat.
4. Elevate the knee. If swelling is present, apply ice or a vinegar compress. Dilute vinegar with water, if you are allergic to vinegar.
5. Rest your knee whenever possible.
6. Use an elastic bandage to provide light compression.

Two simple exercises can give you stronger knees. They help you build stronger thigh muscles and better support for your knees.

1. Sit in a chair with your knees bent, feet flat on the floor. Slowly lift the left foot and extend it straight. Hold it for a count of 10, then lower it slowly. Repeat this 4 to 5 times with the right and left legs for 3 days. Build up to 20 repetitions.
2. If you have a bungie cord or an old fashioned bicycle tube, tie it around the feet of a chair. Now sit comfortably in the chair and slip both feet behind the bungie cord or tube until your feet are pressing against it. Push, one foot at a time, against the rubber, as if you were to extend your knees. Hold the pressure to the count of 6. Relax and repeat with the other leg. After about a week, you should be able to increase your count to 10 for each leg. Do this no more than 6 times for each leg. If your knees hurt, cut back and consult your physician.

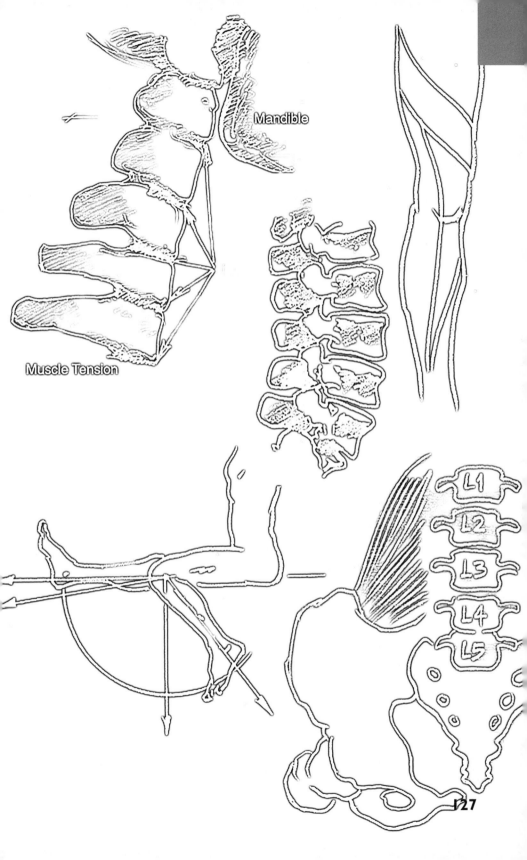

Mandible

Muscle Tension

L1
L2
L3
L4
L5

127

NOW TEST YOURSELF

(Please use a separate sheet of paper.)

1. How is your rib cage held together?

2. How many moves does your ribcage undergo in a single day?

3. What is a hard frame?

4. What is a soft frame?

5. How much do your lungs weigh?

6. What does your viscera consist of?

7. What causes restrictions?

8. Can your ribcage become deformed?

9. How should you inhale?

10. What should you build up besides your muscles?

11. How can you ease pain in your chest?

CHAPTER 11:

THE RIB CAGE

Honor your breath
Honor your heart
And your mind
will follow!
This way
You retain mastery
over yourself!

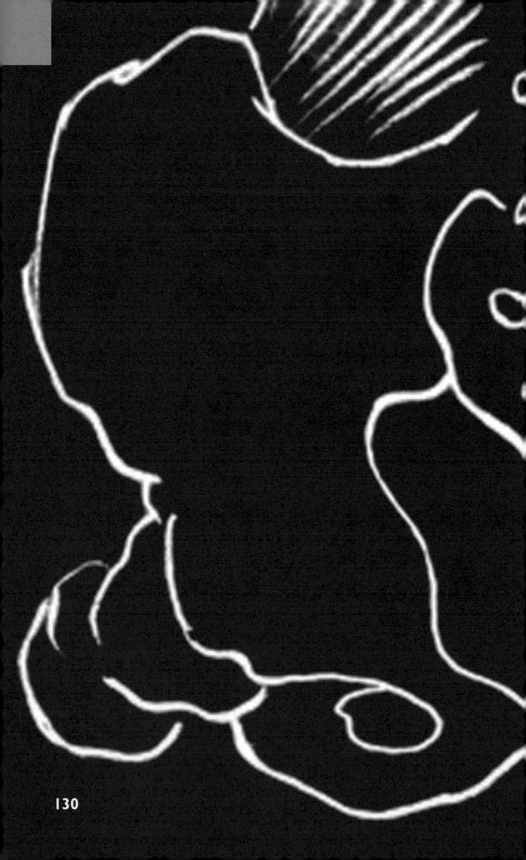

Your rib cage is a hard frame held together by your breast plate (the sternum), ribs, and spine. Believe it or not, this cage has somewhere around 150 articulations, which makes it very flexible. One of your ribs is in contact with six areas (articulations). The average doctor does not pay much attention to five of these articulations. He or she will focus only on the one articulation at the spinal column; yet, most of the trauma is found away from the spine. The reason is simple: You do not breathe only with your spine; you take in oxygen with the entire rib cage. One rib, restricted in its movement, can cause many problems.

Did you know that in a single day, your entire rib cage undergoes more than 3 million moves? Plus, your heart, a key component in rib cage movement, makes over a hundred thousand movements daily. And, you do not have to spend any time directing all these movements. Your conscious mind is much too busy with the world outside, so someone or something is inside you directing these movements.

You have inside this hard frame a soft frame, which consists of fasciae, ligaments, and visceral organs. This fascial system protects the organs inside the hard frame while the frame moves. Because the soft frame is a part of the hard frame, any injury to the hard frame or one of its parts can affect the organs. Did you know that your lungs weigh as much as one and one-third kilograms? This indicates that the soft frame is very strong and thick.

Your visceral frame consists of your heart and lungs. Both of these organs move constantly. Any restriction to your hard frame can cause restriction to the pleura and will affect your respiration.

What causes restrictions?

1.   mechanical problems

2.   infections

3.   tumors

4.   trauma, such as a fall, a blow to the chest or to your shoulder, to your back, of course, and especially to your lower neck where it connects with your rib cage, near your first rib. A lower cervical problem disturbs the pleural system and

upper back fascia.

If you have been involved in an automobile accident and you were wearing a seat belt, most likely you have acquired several rib cage (thoracic) restrictions. These restrictions are not so easy to resolve. The belt may have saved your life, but you will retain the effects for a long time. The rib cage can easily become deformed, but because of its ability to mask the injury the symptoms may show up several years after the accident.

You may have developed lesions on your lungs from pneumonia or T.B., in which case the elasticity of the pleura suffers.

If you had any form of upper back surgery, there will be an imbalance in the mobility of the thoracic frame. This is also true if there was surgery in the pelvic area. These types of surgeries will destabilize the upper back and the whole thorax.

The lungs and the rib cage as well as the entire thorax are subject to numerous types of tumors. In the initial stages, tumors and their symptoms are confused with other less serious diseases. The reason I mention this is so you are aware of your body. Respect it. Help yourself when you are in a position to do so. Cancer develops very slowly. Do not ignore your health. See your physician now and then, please?

YOUR HEART

Some of you may have had open-heart surgery. I had one recently. It is possible that you have experienced pain in your chest, but the pain was not actual cardiac pain. This experience occurred a few weeks after your surgery. What gave you the pain? Simply stated, your body was traumatized from the operation. Your entire thorax has undergone a shock.

Since my operation, I stretch my thorax every day. I exercise the upper part of my body. I should emphasize that I am not stretching my heart, but my thorax. This stretching brings relief from the pain that was caused by the shortening of the muscles of the thorax as a result of surgery.

If I did not stretch, these muscles would continue to shorten more each day. You must keep moving your arms in every direction. Use the doorway or the chinning exercise. Devise your own exercises. You will benefit by them.

The purpose of stretching the thorax is:

1. to release the muscular and fascial system
2. to help your osteoarticular system

Through gradual loosening of the soft tissues, the restrictions in your vertebrae and your rib cage will become obvious. These restrictions should be released by a competent physician, an osteopath, or your chiropractor. Do not attempt to release these restrictions by yourself, with the help of a friend, or your masseur, as your blood pressure needs to be checked before and after the osteoarticular restrictions are tackled.

Please, never take a steam bath followed by immersion in a cool pool or a cold shower soon after. You may damage the muscles of your heart. Heat draws your blood away from your internal organs and from your brain. Chances are that you will cause your brain to become more anemic during this time, and you may experience lightheadedness or dizziness. You surely do not wish to endanger your health, so I suggest that you compromise: take a lukewarm shower, enough to cause your soap to bubble, then cool the water down slowly until it is cold. This will make you feel refreshed. Cold water does not cause peripheral circulatory collapse; hot water and hot steam will.

Use good judgment. Never let hot water hit your chest directly, especially if you have high blood pressure.

Speaking about your heart: Do you drink enough water to keep your blood thin, so that your blood flows more easily? If not, drink a glass of water every hour until your mouth and tongue are moist. Keep this moist feeling in your mouth by drinking several times during the day. You may not love water, but your blood needs it. Drinking water will aid your heart which is working so hard to keep you alive. Water relieves stress on your heart.

Eat foods that contain potassium. Your heart requires it. Your kidneys don't store potassium in your body and each time you pass urine, you lose some potassium. A good source of potassium is found in apple cider vinegar. Honey is also rich in potassium, as are bananas, asparagus, all citrus fruits, and red meat. It is up to you to take care of your heart. Find and eat the foods that promote good health. Also, make sure that your salt intake is minimal. Use salt substitutes or skip it completely; plenty of salt occurs naturally in the healthy foods you eat.

I wonder if you know the facts about blood pressure? You blood pressure is forever changing as a result of the expansion and contraction of your blood vessels, not because of the force of your heart's contractions. The elasticity of your blood vessels is the key. When the arteries are free from tension, they become relaxed and your blood pressure is normal. However, when your arteries are under stress or filled with plaque they are less elastic, and your blood pressure goes up. The best thing you can do to help yourself is to teach yourself to relax. Try the exercise shown here.

Remember, if you keep pressuring your arteries, and if you don't drink enough water, you may cause damage to your internal organs. As I have said: Learn to respect your body and you will learn to respect yourself.

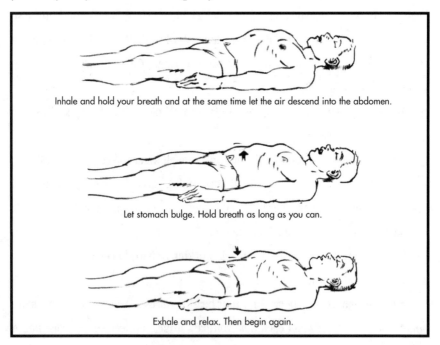

Inhale and hold your breath and at the same time let the air descend into the abdomen.

Let stomach bulge. Hold breath as long as you can.

Exhale and relax. Then begin again.

Master this exercise

INCREASE YOUR ENERGY—BREATHE PROPERLY

When your senses cause you to be lost
When your mind deceives you
Take a deep, deep breath
Then turn to your feelings
They
Will lead you to safety
Feelings—
like your breath—are
never deceived and
will not mislead you.

Your body needs oxygen in order to produce energy. With less oxygen, energy levels are automatically lowered and you feel debilitated. When you are tired and feel lethargic, you are oxygen-starved.

Don't inhale through your mouth; use your nose, which is designed to filter the air before it gets to your lungs. You need to exercise your rib cage and the surrounding muscles required for bringing clean air into your lungs and removing carbon dioxide. If you fail to expand and use these muscles, they will shrink, and they do so slowly and imperceptibly. They will also lose their elasticity and pretty soon you will not be able to take a deep breath.

Everybody can forget how to breathe properly. As you rise from sleep, this is what you do. Don't get out of bed yet.

1. Close your mouth.
2. Relax your abdominal muscles, letting the diaphragm push your stomach down.
3. Relax your body.
4. Now take a deliberately slow breath. Feel the air go down into your abdomen.
5. Hold to the count of four, then exhale.

6. Start over until you have inhaled at least 10-15 deep breaths.

Now you can get up and prepare for your day. Repeat this breathing exercise several times during the day, and you will notice that you do not feel tired. Remember, breath is your life, your sustaining power, the means to maintain good health.

Become active. Activity is your opportunity to strengthen all the organ systems in your body and your mind as well. Remember, motion is the speech of life. Your activity is your speech, giving witness that you are here and you are making a statement about yourself.

We feed our bodies from the fruits of the earth, but we often neglect to take in sufficient amounts of that precious air of heaven. These two in combination will give you all the energy you need for a healthy body and a healthy mind.

Don't fall into the habit of taking the air for granted. The chances are that you don't inhale properly, that you don't take enough air in to exchange the old air in your lungs. The air must be consciously taken deeply into your lungs so that it will invigorate you. Learn to conserve your energy. Do not scatter it. Develop your body through right living and right breathing. Take deep breaths as often as possible during the day.

The fruits of the earth you have to pay for, you have to work for. But the fruit of heaven—the air, oxygen—comes to you free. Learn to heal yourself by practicing love, by smiling, by being good to others and to yourself.

Breathing is life. When you cannot get enough air, when you have difficulty in catching your breath, you know you are in trouble. Therefore, conserve your energy by building up your oxygen reserve in every cell of your body. Learn that pain can be eased by proper breathing. Slow, deep breaths will remove the toxins in your blood, which will help you to overcome pain. Start to breathe:

1. inhale to the count of four

2. hold the breath while you count to four

3. exhale slowly

4. hold your breath to the count of four

Repeat as often as necessary.

5. While inhaling, move your attention away from the area of pain by looking into the palm of one hand or at an imaginary point on the wall or ceiling. This will help. But the breath will do the work as you exchange the stale air in your lungs for fresh air.

Place your palm over the painful area. Breathe and exhale with force through your mouth. Inhale through your nose only. Next, practice the following breathing:

1. Sit or stand with your back slightly curved. Then inhale and tighten your buttocks, your anus, and your perineum. While straightening your neck, draw in your chin.

2. Exhale slowly. Your stomach will flatten.

3. Move the upper part of your abdomen in and out as much as a half a dozen times. Hold your breath while doing this. Now relax and breathe naturally.

4. Repeat, but this time move your navel area six times.

5. Repeat, but move to the lower abdominal area.

This exercise is good for moving your intestines, which become constipated due to sedentary living, prescription medications, insufficient fluid intake, wrong diet, smoking or heavy drinking, or recreational drugs.

You must value your lungs. Learn to care for yourself. Appreciate the talents you have been given. Now learn to breathe with a purpose in mind.

1. I know your hands cannot reach too far behind your back, but place them as far up your back as you can.

2. Inhale, pressing your fingers on your back as close to or on your spine itself, if possible.

3. Exhale and bend backward at the same time. Do this several times.

FATIGUE

When you are exhausted after a hard day's work, or if you are exhausted from emotional stress, or through plain mental exhaustion, place your hands slightly above your lower ribs, and, as you inhale, hold your breath and lightly pump your ribs a couple of times. Then exhale, and repeat three to four times.

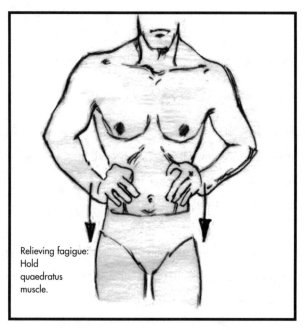

Relieving fagigue:
Hold
quaedratus
muscle.

This exercise will help you if you have pain in your back while walking.

NERVOUS TENSION AND HEADACHE

Tension is usually caused by stress that has been building over a long period of time. Your abdominal area becomes tense, and you may suffer sleepless nights and headaches. You have to relax your spine, especially your spinal cord. Follow these steps for relief:

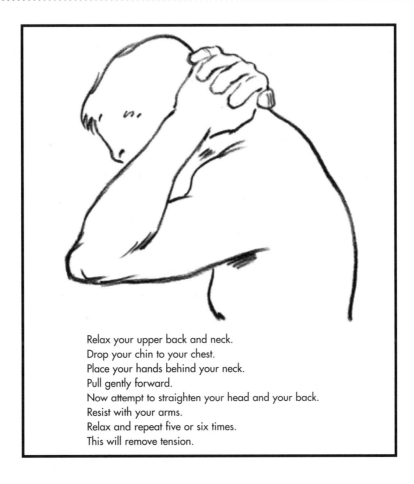

Relax your upper back and neck.
Drop your chin to your chest.
Place your hands behind your neck.
Pull gently forward.
Now attempt to straighten your head and your back.
Resist with your arms.
Relax and repeat five or six times.
This will remove tension.

1. First, press with the palms of your hands the upper abdominal area under your rib cage, near and under your breast plate. While you inhale, hold your palms firmly on the muscles. Hold your breath for about 20 seconds.

2. Exhale and release your hands and let the abdominal muscles resume their normal movements.

3. Move your hands over your navel and repeat this several times.

By now you should know how to take deep breaths. Remember, a knot in your abdomen can cause pain anywhere in your body. Now take off your shoes and your socks or stockings.

1. Start by curling your toes, especially your big toes. Wash your big toe with an ice cube, fast. Do not freeze your toe; just wash it. Soak up the water, but do not rub the toe dry. Slowly, you will feel the nervous tension and headache go away.

2. Next, pick up your socks with your toes. Rest and breathe normally.

3. While you breathe deeply, massage both sides of your nose, then move your hands over your cheekbones, and bring them to your ears, then back to your nose, and repeat a few times. This will relieve the tension in your face.

Nervous tension may be caused by sitting for a long time at a computer or at a desk or over a bench bent over where your neck is under constant strain. This will cause pain in your shoulder muscles and give you a headache. In this case, inhale while you press your tongue firmly against the palate. Extend your neck and exhale, and relax your tongue. This is a quick and easy way to relive tension in your neck. The breath does the work!

RELAX YOUR SPINE

You can relax your spine sitting or standing. If you sit, be sure you are comfortable. Do not allow your back to touch the chair, and make sure to wear loose clothing.

1. Begin by exhaling, letting your arms fall loosely by your side. Let them hang; don't pay any attention to them. Relax.

2. Inhale, and gently let your head fall back as far as it can. Arching your back, push your chest and stomach outward.

3. Hold this position and tighten the muscles of your back.

4. Exhale, and now bring your back forward, rounding your back. Bring your chin down onto your breast plate. Don't tighten any muscles.

Repeat several times.

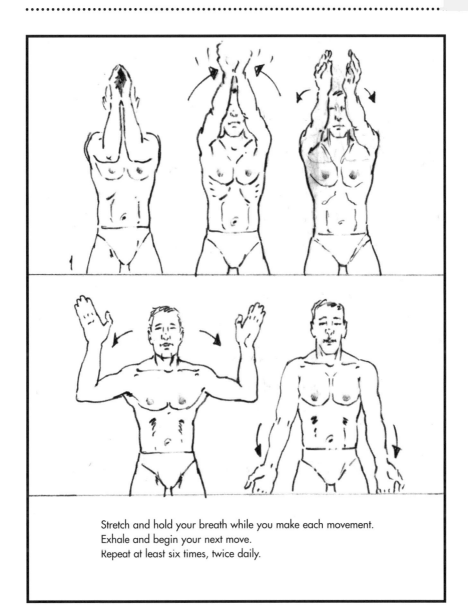

Stretch and hold your breath while you make each movement.
Exhale and begin your next move.
Repeat at least six times, twice daily.

CHAPTER 12 EXAMINATION

NOW TEST YOURSELF

(Please use a separate sheet of paper.)

1. How does emotion affect your health?

2. Can pain be a symbolic manifestation of a problem?

3. Who is the person behind health?

4. Why are you a success?

5. What should you focus your mind on?

CHAPTER 12:

YOUR EMOTIONS

Judgement is the knowing
the how to understand
the language of your own life
and the life of others.
Then
know yourself
before
you know the others!

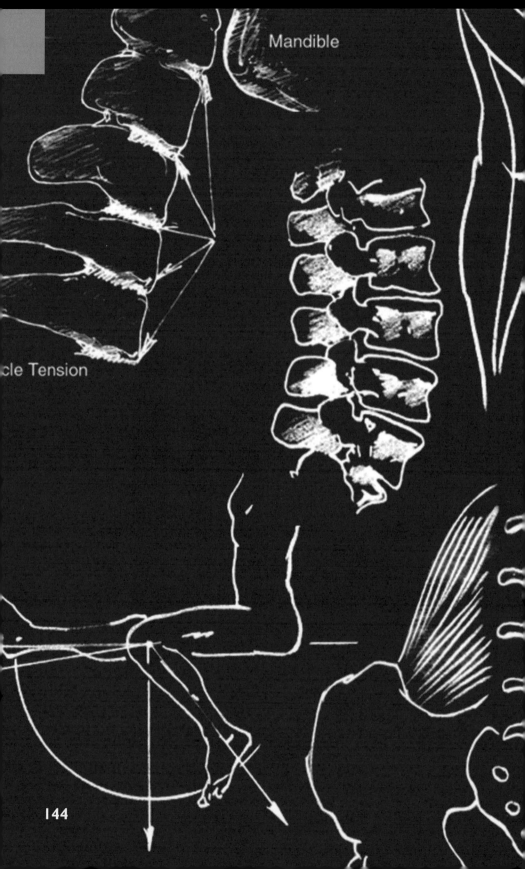

Mandible

cle Tension

144

F aith and truth work hand in hand. Be true to yourself. Be true to your fellow human beings. Be patient! Affirm to yourself that you believe that you can achieve your goals, that you trust in the power and the wisdom of your life— that spark that never fails you.

By now you have realized that your emotions can and do affect your health. Your feelings and thoughts affect your back as well as every organ system in your body.

One of my patients was bent way over and to one side. His head was bent forward to the floor. He said that he had this type of pain for a couple of years. When I won his trust, he revealed that he was undergoing a separation from his wife after 20 years. Any time they had an argument, his back would go into spasm, and he found himself in this same position. After we talked several times, he realized that emotional stress exacerbated a mechanical problem in his spine and his thinking and feeling were being expressed symbolically.

Pain is often a manifestation of an emotional process. We know that emotion can elevate your blood pressure or lower it. Because emotional tension and wrong thinking will damage your health, it is important to realize that you are the power behind your health. Be aware that in your daily living, you alone determine your well being. Manage your emotions consciously and with constructive purpose. Tension damages your heart, your body, and your judgment.

ANXIETY

If you are between 40 and 50 years old, you may have some form of anxiety about your health. Don't worry; almost everyone has the same anxiety. This is commonly called midlife crisis. You may experience some feeling of loss or a feeling that there is not much time left to achieve the goals you set your heart on earlier in life; that your opportunities have narrowed; that you need to change your career, yet you feel unable to compete with younger people. You may feel that your body cannot perform physically as it did before. These feelings are new, and you don't know how to handle them. Tension begins to mount, not just in your mind but in your muscles as well.

It's understandable that you would like to recapture your youth, but you must not try to live backward. The tree cannot be the seed again. You must become a person with inner stability.

1. Tell youself, You are a success. You have reached this, your present age. There are many people much younger than you who will never have this opportunity.

2. Do not become shortsighted, focusing on the past, or on what you have lost.

3. Keep reminding yourself about what you have achieved.

4. Focus on what you may achieve in the future and what you can achieve in the present.

5. Remember, the farmer must each season cultivate his field and tend to his crops each day. He doesn't have time to worry about failures.

6. Do not cultivate tension or fear in any part of yourself.

7. Be positive. Exert yourself. It is never too late.

8. Accept yourself. Accept your age. Accept where you are at this time.

9. Find new ways to improve yourself. Find new hope for your present, and find faith in yourself and your life.

10. Be hopeful about your future.

11. Become the hero of your own life, live fully each day, each moment.
    Faith is the foundation on which health and happiness depends.

FEAR

If you truly wish to help yourself, ask yourself, "What am I afraid of today?" When you have found your answer, then ask yourself, "Why do I avoid facing up to this fear and its cause?" Now write the answer down so that you do not forget it. Face up to the cause of your fear and bring it out into the open so that you can release its hold on you.

Fear cannot be destroyed by will alone. It is an emotion, and you must understand its inner workings. It can work for you or against you—the choice is yours. It is an image of your feelings about yourself, about the world outside of yourself, and of your separation from those who care about you, and, above all, it is a separation from the spark of life within you.

USE WHAT YOU ALREADY KNOW

If you want to grow—to progress—you must always follow your inner judgment, your gut feeling. Your mind may be easily swayed, but not your feelings.

If you put forth the necessary effort you will realize your hopes and your dreams. Remember, the things you dream about are not always easy to attain, but effort and hard work can bring them about, regardless of how long it takes.

- Your experiences are your teachers. Learn from them.
- Refuse to be judged on the basis of your emotional likes or dislikes: Be judged only on your character and on your achievements. Judge yourself as you are responsible for yourself.
- Always trust your own judgment even if your experience tells you otherwise.
- Keep an open mind so that you can grow.
- Keep on learning throughout your life.
- Work for your goals, but do not harm anyone during your quest.
- Be observant.
- Listen to what you hear and hear what you are listening to by abandoning your prejudices. Pay less attention to the way something is being said; hear only what is actually said.

GOOD RULES TO FOLLOW:

1. Do not react too quickly to any emotional situation.
2. Avoid drawing conclusions quickly until you have had a chance to evaluate the situation.
3. Understand all things fully—especially yourself.
4. Cultivate patience!

Know yourself:

5. Have a clear picture of yourself.

6. Know how you feel about yourself.

7. Know your limitations and your weaknesses, and do something about them.

8. Have a healthy self-image.

Trust yourself:

9. Have self-confidence!

10. Trust the decisions you make.

11. Do not lose your judgment in a crisis. Do not panic.

Living in this way will release your muscles from unnecessary tension. Remember, all things are possible in life; their realization comes through your participation in the opportunities all life holds for you.

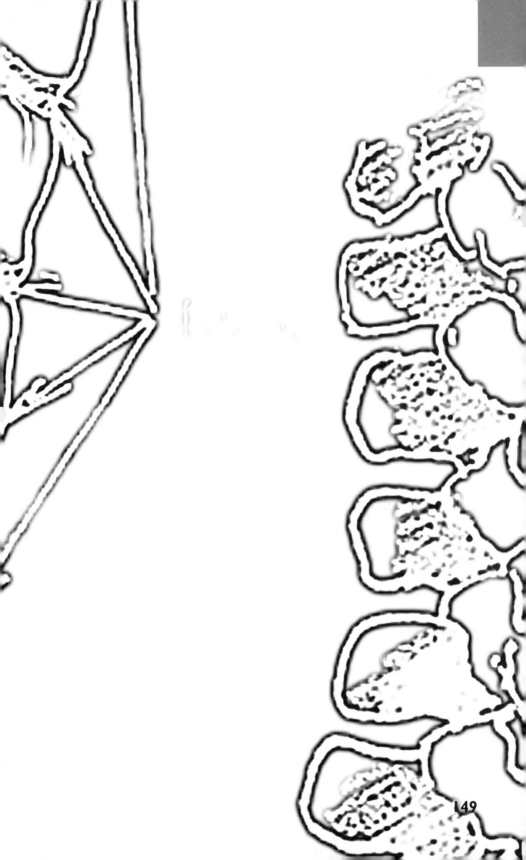

149

CHAPTER 13 EXAMINATION

NOW TEST YOURSELF

(Please use a separate sheet of paper.)

1. Does food have medicinal value?

2. What is onion good for besides food?

3. What is the "other" food you need?

4. Besides food and oxygen, what else do you need?

5. What causes stress?

6. What causes fatigue?

7. What should you consider if you have a pain in a joint?

8. Should you force your spine to perform?

9. What is meant by "normal" weight?

10. Why should you keep your spine supple?

11. What kind of exercise is good for you?

12. Is there a "simple" headache?

13. What happens when your nervous system overworks?

14. What should you avoid?

CHAPTER 13:

FOOD AS MEDICINE

Manage your total self
consciously and with a
constructive purpose.
Find a meaning in each day's
movements around you
As all activity or inactivity
affects you one way or another.

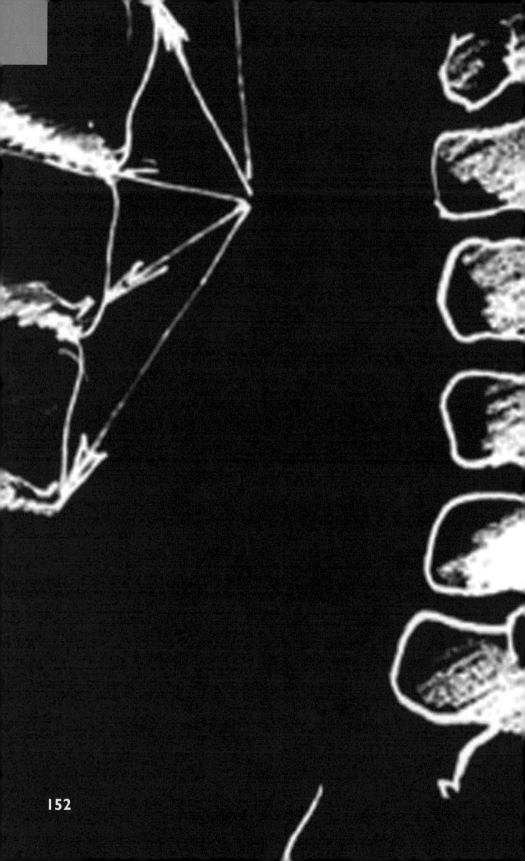

Exercise for emotions

Good food and a healthy environment are proper means to restore emotional balance. Inactivity is a disease in itself. So get moving! Go for a walk. If you are a parent, take your child for a walk. Work out at home or in a park. If you have a yard, play games with your kids. Be active! Put on music and walk, dance, or jump rope.

Eat whole grain food products. Eat several fruits a day. Eat some green leafy vegetables. Eat two servings of protein a day, but do not overeat protein. Drink at least one cup of milk a day. Use sweets and alcohol sparingly, please.

In the beginning of the day or at the end, go for a walk. Do not jog—it destroys your knees and jars your back.

Rule #1 Eat slowly. Do not rush.

Rule #2 Relax after eating at least 15 minutes.

GENERAL RULES

Drink six to eight glasses of water per day.

If you do not suffer from high blood pressure and if you are not restricted to a low sodium diet, have one teaspoon of cider vinegar for potassium or sauerkraut juice daily. Or consume some lemon daily with your meals.

Our bodies are much better suited to treatment with herbal remedies than with isolated chemicals used as prescription medicine. Man's digestive system and his physiology have been adapted to utilize plants as food. These plants have medicinal value besides giving strength to the human body.

Where does the line begin between "food" and "medicine"? Everyone uses lemons and onions, or buys a papaya once in a while, and many eat oats for breakfast or make oatmeal cookies. Did you know that these foods are also medicines? Lemon improves resistance to infections. It contains Vitamin C which is effective against colds and the flu. It also is a preventative for infections of the stomach and thickening of the arterial walls, and it can be used as an antirheumatic, antioxidant, and to reduce fever.

Papaya is a digestive agent used to expel worms. In Latin America, its leaves are used as meat tenderizers. The latex from the trunk of the papaya tree is used externally to heal wounds, boils, and even tumors.

Onion relieves bronchial infections. Onions have been used to treat stings from bees, spiders, and other insects, and to relieve cold symptoms. It has been used as a diuretic, anti-inflammatory, analgesic, and antirheumatic. Onions are eaten all over the world to relieve colds and coughs. Onions are also used in Europe for chest pains and also to prevent respiratory and oral infections. In the town where I was born, onions were used to stop earaches by warming the juice and dropping it into the ear. My father used it to drain pus from sores. And the peasants used onions as an aphrodisiac as well as a hair growth stimulant.

Some of the vegetables and fruits you use daily have medicinal properties. Here are just a few examples.

FOOD	MEDICINAL USE
Garlic	respiratory infections: To relieve nose and throat infections as well as chest congestion; anti-fungal: cardiovascular benefits, lowers blood pressure and cholesterol. *Beware! It slows blood clotting by keeping blood platelets from clumping. Don't take it with cumadin or aspirin, ticlid or plavix.*
Cayenne; chili	aids indigestion; a warming stimulant
Radish	In the mustard family, it has been applied as a poultice to painful joints

Celery	a mild diuretic. The seeds have been used to relieve arthritic pains and as an antispasmodic.
Cinnamon	for common colds; for digestive problems; as an antiviral
Clove	analgesic; prevents vomiting; antispasmodic; eliminates parasites
Avocado	treatment for diarrhea; expels worms; relieves coughs; promotes menstrual flow
Corn (silk)	used to treat urinary conditions and help reduce blood pressure
Ginger	to relieve digestive difficulties caused by motion sickness and morning sickness; nausea, especially if receiving chemotherapy. *Beware! It should not be taken with anti-clotting drugs such as cumadin, ticlid or plavix.* helps blood circulation; inhibits coughing
Pineapple	aids indigestion; contains Vitamin A and C; reduces excessive gastric acid
Asparagus	a laxative and diuretic
Carrot	stimulates urine; supports the liver; improves night blindness and general vision; carotene is converted to Vitamin A by the liver; relieves gassy colic. (Caution for women who are pregnant: Do not use carrot seeds, which may be abortifacient.)
Apricot	mild laxative

Potato	helpful when taken in moderation for relief from acidity and pain from ulcers. Mashed pulp has been used to relieve painful joints, headaches, and even backaches.
Ginseng	increases energy and stamina. *Beware! May increase blood sugars, if you are a diabetic or a borderline diabetic. Consult your physician before taking it. It may interfere with anti-clotting drugs.*
Grapefruit	Contains Vitamin C. *If taking cholesterol medication, beware! Grapefruit raises blood levels of some cholesterol medications and might increase muscle pain or produce weakness, signals of muscle breakdown.*
Licorice	treats colds, coughs and respiratory infections. *Beware! It depletes your body's potassium. Do not combine with lenoxin. The potassium loss could disrupt the rhythm of your heart. And, if on a diuretic, it can further deplete potassium.*

Become aware of what you eat and what foods can do for you, and how you can use food as medicine. It is obvious to many today that the quality of your diet is essential in maintaining and regaining good health. I am not a dietician, nor will I tell you exactly what you should eat except to urge you to use good judgment, as you become what you absorb from what you eat.

The other nourishment that you need is oxygen. Herbs can help to relax the bronchial muscles and stimulate respiration.

Good health needs a balanced nervous system. Your nervous system does not work in isolation but with your endocrine system, which regulate your hormones, including your sex hormones which regulate not just fertility but your vitality and your moods as well. Your nervous system also works in close relationship with your immune system, which resists infections and helps you to recover from illness or injury.

Your body's ability to adapt to the world outside of itself, while all internal systems work in complete harmony, is known as homeostasis.

My purpose in this chapter is to make you knowledgeable about your body's needs. Educate yourself by doing some research about food. Read about foods and how they influence you physically, mentally, and emotionally. Try to eat naturally.

Remember, what you eat and what you weigh is important to you in the long run. The reasons are obvious. Being overweight can increase your risk for heart disease and other major health problems. While I was in practice, I always advised my patients not to follow any particular diet. Instead, I told them they should eat sensibly, exercise, and most importantly, change old habits of indulgence. This is a must in the discipline of staying healthy.

Try not to concentrate on losing weight but on eating right. This is what I recommend:

1. Eat plenty of fruits and vegetables.
2. Be physically active.
3. Maintain a low salt intake.
4. Have sufficient calcium in your diet. Younger women seldom get enough calcium. You need more calcium between birth and your mid-thirties, as your bones develop during this period. Bone density begins to decrease after 35, sometimes earlier. Therefore, drink at least two cups of milk daily, or eat two to three cups of yogurt, or about 8 oz. of cheese per day to prevent osteoporosis. (Do not consume all these in one day!)

5. This is to remind you of #2. You cannot create or restore your bones to good health (proper density) without putting stress on them through exercise. Lift up a chair in the kitchen. Walk in place. Run in place. Jump up and down. Move!

6. Walk in the sun for a few minutes a day. Fifteen or twenty minutes will give your body enough vitamin D. If you cannot do this, be certain to eat enough dairy products.

7. Protein builds bones. If you are a vegetarian, eat soy products or beans. Sesame seeds are also a good source of protein.

8. If you are dieting, realize that if you fail to take in enough calories, your body will start using your own stored protein and you may become protein deficient. If you have a small frame, you are more prone to develop osteoporosis sooner. Extra weight in the form of muscle makes stronger bones.

9. Eat the right variety of foods and you will be healthy. Try to eat foods that will not easily convert to fat, such as sugar and white flour, which stimulate the overproduction of insulin. These foods will make you tired and will set you on a roller-coaster course. The energy they create is fleeting; you are hungry again soon and gaining weight is the end result.

10. Do not weaken your body so that your bones become brittle. Broken bones can become deformity and disability.

WHAT SHOULD BE YOUR WEIGHT GOAL?

Try to weigh what your best weight was at half your present age. For the sake of discussion, if you are now 50, if your best weight was somewhere around age 25, aim for it. Of course, if your best weight is at your present age, try to maintain it.

You cannot discount your genes, which are somewhat responsible for your weight, just as they are for your shape and the color of your eyes. At the same time, you can't blame everything on those genes. Your lifestyle has a great deal to do with what you weigh.

1. Avoid living a sedentary existence.

2. Avoid carrying your weight around your waist and your stomach; these increase your chances of cancer, heart disease, and diabetes.

Focus your attention on changing your present ways of eating, not on losing weight. What does your success depend on? You! Make the effort to walk instead of drive. Swim. If you don't have a swimming pool, lie down on the floor and pretend to swim. Keep active. Put on some good music and dance, or go ride a bicycle. Avoid becoming flabby.

Above all else, enjoy what you eat, and be glad that you can do it!

1. Don't sit down to eat while you are angry or upset about something.

2. Don't air your problems, whatever they are, at the table. A dining table is for meals and family get-togethers, not for arguments.

3. Remember that you need the warmth of your friends and those who love you around you while you eat.

4. Limit what you eat; at the same time, don't eliminate the foods you like.

5. If you are bored during the day, please don't comfort yourself by eating. Food is not a substitute for companionship. Don't twiddle your thumbs. Go for a walk; meditate; but don't fall asleep. Listen to the news, to music. Take an interest in yourself, in your surroundings. Lend a hand to someone who needs what you can offer.

DON'T COUNT CALORIES

Calorie counting will stop you from enjoying what you do eat. Don't skip any meals during the day, especially breakfast. Skipping meals will not cause you to lose those pounds; on the contrary, your metabolism may slow down if you abstain from eating for long periods of time.

Please discard the following excuses from your vocabulary: "I don't have time to eat." "I have to run." "I am late for work." "I am late for a meeting." "I overslept." I am in a rush."

Please accept this last advice. You have judgment. Use it—it is good judgment! Life bestowed it on you! Remember, be yourself! Do not try to be like someone else. Do not imitate. Life made only one of you! Accept yourself as life already has. Remember, you become what you put into yourself, and what you feel about yourself— not what others think about you.

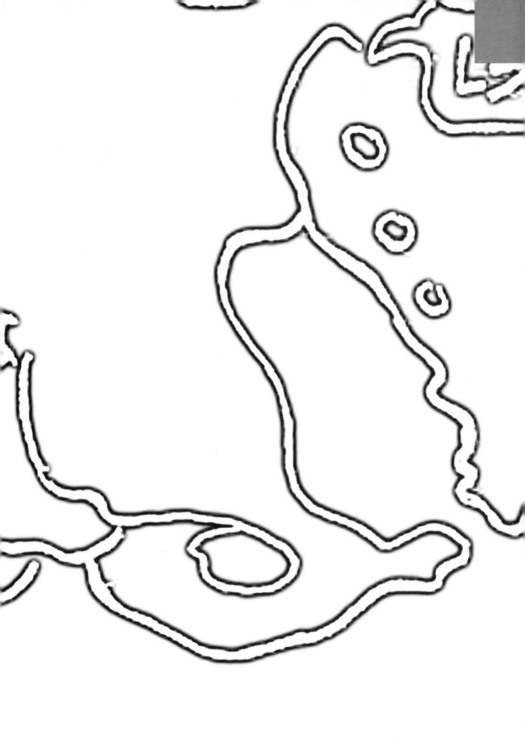

CHAPTER 14 EXAMINATION

NOW TEST YOURSELF

(Please use a separate sheet of paper.)

1. When you have pain and it is not due to a lesion, where should you look?

2. What will restore a muscle to its normal length?

3. What does "myalgia" mean to you?

4. What is a "spasm"?

5. Who is responsible for taking care of your muscles?

6. What kind of pain can your muscles cause?

7. What pain conditions should you be aware of?

8. In which muscle do infants develop tenderness?

9. Should you use heat on trigger points?

10. What is the difference between pain originating in a muscle and pain originating from nerve involvement?

11. What causes weakness suddenly?

12. What does healing depend upon?

CHAPTER 14:

PAIN

One moment of failure
is not a complete one.
But
the denial of that one moment
is.
Learn to accept yourself
as you are.
Then begin your own rebuilding
by expanding your horizons.

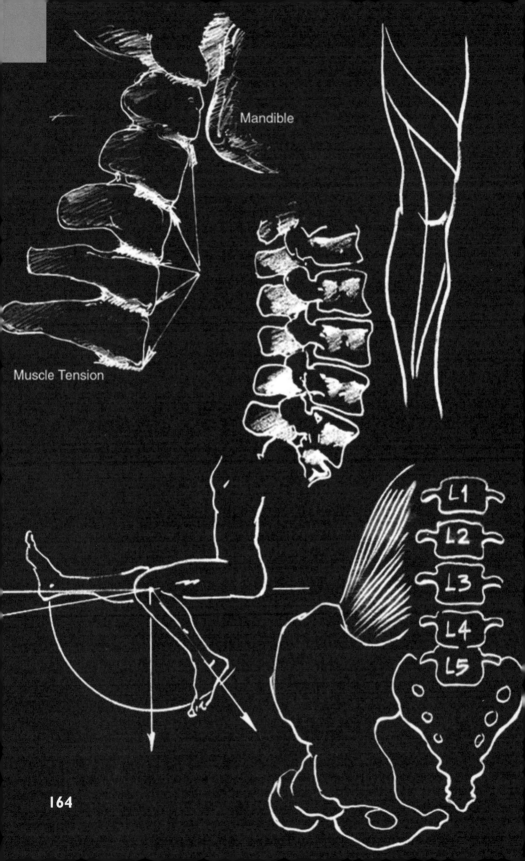

Mandible

Muscle Tension

L1
L2
L3
L4
L5

Take Control of Your Pain

1. The first step toward overcoming pain is to accept it.

2. Do not blame others for your pain, or for not being able to help you to alleviate it. This may not be possible sometimes. It may be necessary to bear that pain for longer than you expect.

3. Do not blame yourself for the pain. The last thing you need at this time is a guilt trip. Having pain is enough of a burden.

> *Blame is the road*
> *that ultimately leads*
> *to devastation and chaos.*

4. When you accept your pain you begin to gain mastery over it, and then you can take steps to overcome it.

5. Pain is friend, a symptom, and a part of everyone's experience. Pain tells you that your body has been wronged, by injury or by disease; that you are in a state of suffering; that it has affected your thinking and your communication with others; that you are, after all, a human being, needing someone more powerful, stronger than yourself to help you.

> *Always understand in yourself*
> *The cause of your pain and your anguish first,*
> *in order that you may be able to understand*
> *the pain others feel, and help them in*
> *overcoming the cause.*

Do Not Divide Yourself

When you have a medical problem you go to a specialist. You see your internist for common problems, a cardiologist for heart problems, a psychiatrist for your mental health. For your moral pain you see your minister, your priest, a rabbi or an iman. But, pain comes to consciousness from various sources. Such as:

- Expectations which you could not fill, imposed by yourself or others
- Low self-esteem
- Guilt
- Fear
- Disease or imbalance in your internal organs
- Hormonal imbalance
- Old injuries
- Parents, children, or siblings against one another
- Forms of injustice
- Pain inflicted by yourself on yourself or on others, physically or emotionally

Now that you know this you have pain and you cannot stop it, what should you do? Keep control over it. Do not hand it over to anyone to solve it.

Wherever your thought goes
so goes your spirit.

REVIEW OF PAIN

1. Pain is a symptom, a friend.
2. When pain is acute—if limited in duration—you usually know its cause.
3. When pain is chronic (it lasts longer than 12 weeks) its cause is more difficult to understand.
4. Pain nerves come from extremes of cold or heat and trauma.
5. Pain comes from inflammation, a process that fights infection. (This is damage control.)
6. Muscle pain is due to spasm or tightness. When you take a muscle relaxant to eliminate your pain, remember that these work primarily in your brain.

All deeds pursue
the soul
as friends or avengers.

7. Stress is a form of pain and pain is a form of stress. Each influences your body. These two, in time, can become chronic.

Resist the temptation to cause
strife or stress.

8. Respond to your pain by focussing your mind on what your body tells you. Such as saying something loud that you can hear: "I hurt! But I can help myself. I will make it! Hold on!" or by counting "one, two, three," and so on.

9. Focus your attention on your breath. You will notice that your breathing may be shallow or disrupted. Bring it under control by breathing more deeply. Tension, stress, and prolonged anxiety cause disruptions in your breathing. Take control by breathing slowly. Use your abdomen and breathe in and out. Deep breaths allow your diaphragm to massage your heart and your intestines.

10. Pace yourself. Do not exhaust your mind or your body. When your body isn't in a state of constant tension, it has a better chance of recuperating. Do not be shy; ask someone to assist you. Know when to limit your activities and know when to increase your activities.

11. Follow the exercises I have outlined to relieve stress. Keep your head high and your body will follow. Smile as much as possible without feeling idiotic— just enough to lift up your spirit.

Let life become
your teacher
and you its fit companion!

12. Exercise for health and well-being. If you have a bicycle, use it. Make sure you go for a walk outdoors. (*Walking on a treadmill may be hard on your back.*) Don't forget to enjoy your life. Become involved with your surroundings, with your neighbors, with your church, mosque or temple. Engage in pleasurable activities. Do not isolate yourself from the world around you.

13. Understand your feelings so you know your pain and its origin. Understand what goes on inside of your body. When you talk to yourself, are you speaking in a way that destroys your self-confidence? Or are you uplifting yourself? Visualize yourself being inside the eye of a storm and slightly above it. Observe your feelings without being affected by them. Remember, your understanding carries the healing power you need.

> *Only in the night*
> *can the stars shine.*

14. Challenge yourself constantly. Remain in control of yourself and you will remain in control of your pain.

> *Be alive and declare it!*
> *The result: liberty to self*
> *in experiencing yourself!*

15. Do not feel helpless because of your pain. Helplessness is an acquired feeling. Never give it power over yourself. Do not blame anyone for your pain or your suffering. Examine your role in the reason for your pain. This must happen before you hope to overcome it.

16. Develop an optimistic outlook and a non-judgmental attitude toward your fellow human beings. They, too, have problems; they, too, have pains and feelings like yourself.

17. See yourself in a positive way. Develop a sense of humor about the world. This does not mean that you will be pain-free, but the pain will be less powerful over you.

It is more painful to live
a life of illusion
than that of reality.

18. Don't work longer than an hour at your desk at a time. Take deep breaths while you sit at your desk. Move your eyes around the office to relax them. Blink several times to moisturize your eyes.

19. Move your shoulders forward and backwards. Shake your hands and your arms. Check your back. Make sure you sit erect. Get up and walk around. Move your legs. Move your whole body to stimulate circulation.

20. Have respect for yourself and others will respect you.

POSTURE

Long periods of sitting, typing, talking on the telephone, using the computer will roll your shoulders forward. Your head will feel heavy and you will start forming a hunched back. You want to counteract this feeling. You want to be stretched. You want to grow a little taller.

Your spine needs to be relieved from this unnatural posture. Therefore, do the following:

1. Move your buttock forward in your chair. Sit at the edge. Turn away from your desk. Place your feet flat on the floor, feet and shoulders wide. Sit as straight as you can. Hold your arms in front of your chest, elbows not rigid, palms facing the floor. Take a few deep breaths. At the same time, elevate both shoulders toward the ceiling, moving them up and down several times. Now relax. Begin to move your stomach in and out as you breath in and out.

2. Maintain this position, arms in front of your chest. Inhale and, as slowly as possible, elevate your arms above your head. Keep your eyes slightly toward the ceiling, not level. Your back will slowly give up its forward bend. Hold your breath as long as you can, then exhale bringing your outstretched arms slightly backward, without force. Inhale again and slowly bring your arms in front of you. Begin again. Do this exercise as often as you can. This will help you prevent bad posture and low feelings. At the end of the day you will not feel drained.

YOUR ACHES AND PAINS

In thinking about pain, consider the duration of your present symptoms. How many episodes of pain have you had in your past? How intense is your present pain? How anxious are you about it? Are you depressed from it? How do you rate your health? Poor, satisfactory, good, excellent, or just fair? Are you satisfied with your job? Do your symptoms cause you to be disabled? Do you believe that you should not work with your current pain or symptoms? Do you believe that any physical activity will worsen your pain? Do you believe that normal physical activity is all right for you? Can you tolerate work for at least an hour, maybe two? Can you sleep at night?

Don't think of your pain as something you can't do anything about. Consider the following: If you have pain in any one of your joints, especially in your toe, have your doctor test for gout, which indicates a high level of uric acid in the blood. With proper treatment gout pain can be relieved. Consider a test for rheumatoid arthritis. Chiropractic adjustment will afford you much relief. Take vitamins as supplements.

Remember the organs in your body need nerves from your spine to help them function. Your organs must have an unimpaired nerve supply to them, therefore you must keep your spine supple and loose.

1. Stretch the spine by dangling from an overhead bar. This will make your arms strong. They will support your body weight. Relax your back and your shoulders. Do this for a week. You can swing your legs from side to side. Take your time.

2. Lie down on your back on the bed or on a padded surface. Raise your feet 90 degrees from the floor. Use your arms and hands to support your hips. Take

your time. Inhale as you lift your legs. Hold your breath as long as you can, then lower your legs and exhale. Do this 3 or 4 times, no more.

Exercise will make your muscles elastic, and, as you inhale, your arteries and veins will become elastic as well. Your arteries have muscles as well. Exercise them. Don't wait. Do it every day.

Your spine is different from any other person's. No one moves like you do. It's like your fingerprints. Never force your spine to move the way someone else thinks you should move it. The small muscles of your spine and all the ligaments need time to stretch properly, and they will stretch according to your physiological and mechanical capabilities.

Avoid heavy lifting, especially in the gym, or you may cause hairline fractures of the spine/vertebrae. Never lift more than your own weight, as you may compress the vertebrae of your spine. Remember, your bones can fracture if you use poor judgement. Small abuses of the spine can later lead to arthritis, pain, and limited mobility.

You can help yourself deal with most of your back pains, at least the ones which are muscular in origin. Find any exercise that gives you relief, which means that you correct an imbalance in any tense muscles. Any exercise that helps you to correct this imbalance will help your back. Muscle tension may indicate high levels of stress. Be attentive to your way of living. Do not let your problems become pain.

Please don't run to the surgeon to get rid of back pain before you have exhausted every other means of treatment available. Your pain may not come from a problem that can be seen on an x-ray. Decades of experience have taught me that surgery was seldom needed to relieve back pain.

With a little help, the body can adjust to everything, even what is known as a disc problem. Within your body is a physician that creates health and the medicine it needs. Visit your doctor, chiropractor, or osteopath to relieve you from any mechanical malposition in your spine. It is also possible that post-surgical conditions may create pain. Many of my patients had two to five surgeries on the back to relieve their pain but results were usually disappointing. If surgery is needed, a good surgeon will tell you honestly that surgery is a risk. The failure is often not the surgeon's fault; pain may not be physiological but symbolic!

WHAT CAN YOU DO TO GET RID OF YOUR PAIN?

All healing is but a release
from the illusion of the past.
Past fears—past pains
To hold on to these
will prevent any happiness in the present.

Examine your way of life. See what and who you resent. Write it down; do not keep it inside. Who do you hate? And why? Are you bored?

Having done this and determined that your aches and pains are not symbolic in origin, you are ready for the following: Ask someone to help you. First, take a marking pencil. Lie down on your stomach on a bed. Have your helper press with palms down on your back and, with his/her fingers, find your painful area. See if pressure will create pain in some other part of your body. Mark the skin where the referred pain manifests and begin to stretch the muscles slowly and gently. Do not rub or press hard. Stretch for 10 to 15 seconds in each area; more than that will irritate the tissue. When you are in pain your nervous system becomes overactive, and your pain receptors oversensitive, so your pain becomes magnified. Even if you block out pain through visualization, the effect on the nervous system remains.

The overactive nervous system requires more energy. When muscles and nerves are overactive; the body is in an increased state of tension which causes fatigue. Pain and physical exhaustion go hand-in-hand. When you are in pain, you are fatigued;

when you are fatigued, you have pain somewhere, if not in your body, then in your mind or somewhere in your life.

An aspirin may temporarily relieve the pain, but not the cause of the pain. Medication to prevent exhaustion and overactivity of the nervous system is fine, but only occasionally.

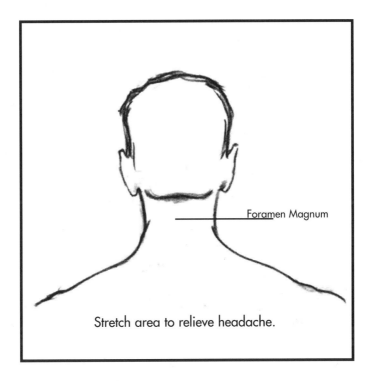

Foramen Magnum

Stretch area to relieve headache.

HEADACHES

Peace is the savior of the mind
and the human mind does
indeed need peace.

There is no such thing as a simple headache that has no cause. I will show how you can help yourself temporarily until you discover the reason for your headache.

1. When you first notice the headache lie flat on your back. Do not sit in a chair; lie on a firm surface. Do not put a pillow under your head; your head must be on the same level as the rest of your body.

2. Elevate both hands above your shoulders. Bend your elbows and place the middle fingers of each hand at the base of the skull. Stretch your neck a little. This will allow your fingers to slip into an opening (groove) called "Foramen Magnum" (the "great opening" formed at the base of your skull where the head and neck meet). Place your fingers in the groove so that both fingertips meet. Bend your knees slightly.

3. Use gentle pressure on the groove and spread the muscles sideways, right finger toward the right ear, left finger to the left ear. Stretch the muscles sideways as if you were pulling a string on an instrument. This will release a lot of the tension that may have contributed to your headache.

4. Repeat several times and you will discover how quickly you can help yourself. If your headache persists, you should have a complete physical examination. Do not use this technique after an accident or a fall in case you may have displaced a vertebrae in your neck. This exercise offers relief for simple tension headaches only.

   Another simple exercise to relieve tension is to take time to be observant during the day. Take several breaks. Look at yourself in a mirror and see who is looking back at you. What is the image saying to you? Now look at your hands and feet, close your eyes and know and feel that your physical body is a part of you and you are its director. Your body carries out your wishes and your desires, both the good and the bad ones. Now relax each part of your body. Open your eyes and look into the mirror and see how your expression has changed. Take a few deep breaths, drink some water, and resume your daily activity. Do this each day and before long you may become better acquainted with yourself. What you will learn is what you don't know that can and needs to be discovered by you every day.

MUSCLE PAIN

Muscle pain that is referred to various parts of the body has been overlooked in the treatment of aches and pains. In my practice I found relief of this kind of pain particularly necessary to help my patients return to their comfortable life.

When you experience pain that does not originate in a lesion, a subluxation, or in a symbolic transfer from a life situation, it is a concentration of excessive irritation in a muscle and/or its fascia that is expressed as a symptom in the movement of a muscle. This irritation causes tenderness in the muscle and prevents extension to its normal length. In other words, the muscle becomes shorter and weaker. Stretching the muscle and relaxing it will help restore the muscle to its normal length.

The word "myalgia" has two meanings: one refers to aching muscles due to disease, such as an infection caused by a virus; the second refers to tenderness of a muscle or group of muscles caused by excessive irritation. Do not confuse the meanings. You have also heard the word "spasm." It is an increased tension which may cause your muscle to shorten due to non-voluntary motor activity. A spasm cannot be stopped by your willing a muscle to relax. A spasm is not a contracture, which is an abnormal shortening of muscle tissue that makes the muscle resistant to passive stretching.

You have 696 muscles: 347 paired and 2 unpaired muscles. This does not include heads, bellies, and other parts of muscles. Your voluntary muscles (skeletal) account for over 40% of your body weight. All of these muscles are capable of developing "trigger points," producing pain and other distressing symptoms at a distant location in your body. A trigger point is a firm hard "ropy" muscle in spasm.

The average physician pays very little attention to your muscles. He or she may tell you to take a "muscle relaxant," and your problem is supposed to be solved. A competent chiropractic doctor or an osteopath will pay attention to your muscles, but the responsibility of taking care of your muscles is in your hands.

175

Pain in your muscles can cause stiffness, and your motion will become restricted. The symptoms you may experience range from being painless in motion, even if the motion is restricted such as in a very old person, to being incapacitated by agonizing pain. While pain in your muscles is never life threatening, it can cause a diminished quality of life. Muscle pain can cause headaches, pain in your shoulders, and pain in your lower back. If you neglect the warning signs, the pain may become chronic.

Analgesics are palliative. They never remove the cause. You can suppress the real cause of your pain unless you are aware of the following conditions:

1. If your muscles ache over a period of 8-12 weeks
2. If you have persistent tenderness in several areas of your body
3. If your skin is tender over your shoulders and shoulder blades
4. If you are restless and cannot find a comfortable way to sleep, and if when you rise you are stiff and tired, don't wait! Seek help! But to prevent this from happening to you, take cool showers as often as you can. Avoid hot showers and hot baths; heat is harmful. These will cause your muscles to stiffen when they cool.

Your normal muscles do not contain any trigger points. They have no taut muscle fibers causing tenderness. They cannot be made to twitch. Above all, they do not send out pain signals when they are pressed. If you are a sedentary person and middle-aged, you are a candidate to develop trigger points. And, if you are female and elderly, you are more likely to develop muscle pain of myofascial type #2 (excessive irritation in the muscles.) But luckily women tend to seek treatment much sooner than men!

Infants have muscle tenderness in their abdominal muscles primarily in the straight muscle (rectus abdominis), which gives them colic. These are easily relieved by a vapor coolant applied over the muscle, which helps to inactivate the myofascial trigger point. In children I have found the most common pain was myofascial pain, caused by trigger points which, if not treated early in childhood, come back, haunting adulthood and old age. Paradoxically, activity increases the pain, but activity also stretches the muscles, which can reduce pain.

As activity decreases with age, pain lessens, but muscles become shorter and shorter and stiffen. Limited motion is then the norm. Yet, all this can be prevented if you learn to use ice to treat the trigger point. Wash the trigger point and surrounding tissue with ice; let it melt. This way you do not freeze the area but rather bring circulation to that area. The pain-causing trigger point becomes weaker and weaker as you regularly apply ice over the point. The muscle will no longer remember the pain as it lengthens and relaxes. The discomfort will also disappear and eventually you will be pain free.

Pain originating from a trigger point is not the same type of pain that comes from nerve involvement. All trigger points are activated by overwork, by becoming fatigued and overloading your muscles, by a trauma, or by catching cold in your muscles. Trigger points can also be activated by disease in your body or in your joints, by distressed emotions, ulcers, heart problems such as myocardial infarction, kidney problems, kidney stones, or colic.

You must also remember that you cannot always depend on your muscle strength! Weakness can set in suddenly; you might drop things; your legs may give out under you; your grip may weaken and you will not be able to hold on to things; you may fall. Weakness that comes on suddenly results from the body's reaction to prolonged inactivity, the resulting muscle weakness, and the body's attempt to protect the muscle from a painful contraction.

Fear tears like a lion
the mind of man
peace delivers.

. . . .

COMMON CHRONIC PAIN CONDITIONS

Neck and low back:

Difficult to diagnose when they become chronic. Remember that the spine is always in an unstable state, so seek help from a competent healthcare provider.

Fibromyalgia:

This is a chronic pain syndrome. Women are more affected than men. It has many names—"fibrositis," "myofascial pain," "viral syndrome," "fatigue syndrome."

Headaches:

Many factors contribute to headaches, such as coffee, aspirin, other anti-inflammatory medications, muscle tension, T.M.J. (Temporo-Mandibular Joint strain: grinding teeth or clenching jaw), fasting (especially among those who suffer from low blood sugar).

Cystitis:

Inflammation of the bladder, mostly in women.

Diabetes-caused neuropathy:

A pathologic change in the outer nervous system aggravated by the disease.

Post-operative neuralgia:

A functional disturbance of the outer nervous system due to surgical trauma.

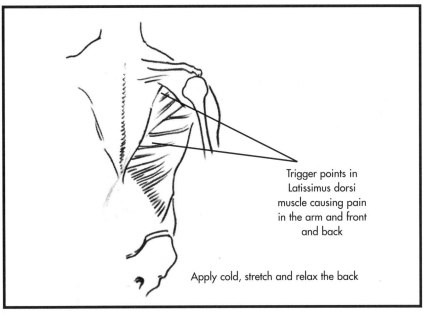

Trigger points in
Latissimus dorsi
muscle causing pain
in the arm and front
and back

Apply cold, stretch and relax the back

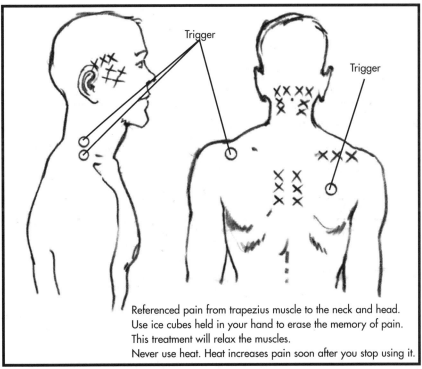

Trigger

Trigger

Referenced pain from trapezius muscle to the neck and head.
Use ice cubes held in your hand to erase the memory of pain.
This treatment will relax the muscles.
Never use heat. Heat increases pain soon after you stop using it.

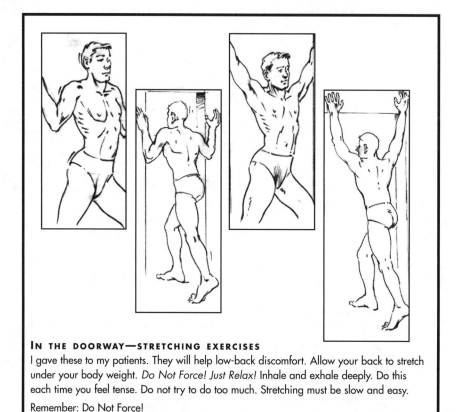

IN THE DOORWAY—STRETCHING EXERCISES
I gave these to my patients. They will help low-back discomfort. Allow your back to stretch under your body weight. *Do Not Force! Just Relax!* Inhale and exhale deeply. Do this each time you feel tense. Do not try to do too much. Stretching must be slow and easy.
Remember: Do Not Force!

HOW TO FIND A TRIGGER POINT

1. When a trigger point is present, stretching of any kind increases pain.

2. If stretching the muscle to its full length increases pain, seek help or apply cold immediately.

3. If the range of motion is restricted it means that the taut band will not permit the muscle to extend to its full range.

4. Applying pressure with your fingers causes the muscle to jump.

5. Sustained pressure on a trigger point intensifies pain.

6. A blood test shows no abnormalities or significant changes attributable to trigger points, e.g., a clot.

7. Electromyographic examination of muscle reveals no abnormalities.

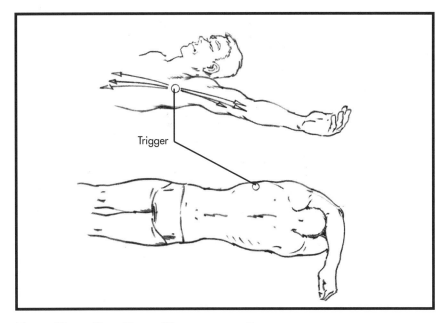

Trigger

TIME WILL NOT HEAL MYOFASCIAL PAIN

Healing depends upon eliminating the trigger point and its causes in the over-irritated muscle or muscles. If you treat a trigger point by cold, the response will be noticeable. The tenderness and twitching disappears, and muscle tensions are released; restricted motion is alleviated.

For lasting relief seek the aid of a reliable doctor, a chiropractor, or an osteopath. When you use ice, stretch the affected muscle. Use less ice, rather than more, as excessive cooling tends to aggravate rather than relax. Release of tension in the muscle through cooling and stretching will be noticeable when motion in the affected area is increased.

Now that you know the signs of trigger points, this should help you to evaluate what action to take to remain healthy and happy.

LIFTING

Hernias are protrusions of an organ or tissue through a weakened abdominal wall. If you experience the onset of a hernia while you are lifting something, do not wait. Pay attention to it: Hernias require immediate treatment to prevent possible strangulation of the intestines. A hernia is recognizable by the following signs:

1. a lump, usually in the groin, or near the umbilical area
2. pain or discomfort in the area of the hernia
3. coughing brings on pain
4. lifting something heavy brings on pain
5. standing for a long time brings on pain

Hernias can happen without warning. If your body becomes weak through illness, you are more susceptible to hernias as the walls of your abdomen are weak. Males are most likely to have a hernia in the inguinal area because there is a space in the groin area that remains unsupported after the testicle descends into the scrotal sac. I offer the following suggestions:

1. Use your hands and your feet as levers when lifting.
2. When you lift something from the floor, begin to balance yourself with your toes. Your big toes are designed to support this action.
3. Next, lower your weight onto your heels, where most of your weight should be.
4. Your knees should be bent and your spine straight. As you start lifting, push with your knees downward, hands firm on the object to be lifted.
5. Elevate the object to a comfortable level, while straightening your legs. Now you can move the object.
6. Remember: Inhale as you lift. Exhale in the erect position. Hold your breath while you carry the object. This will protect you from injury. If you exhale while lifting, you may injure your back.
7. Avoid carrying an object even as light as a book with your palms in the upward position (open handed). Tennis elbow pain can occur, even if you do not play tennis!

CHAPTER 15:

THINGS TO KNOW

One moment of failure
is not a complete one.
But
the denial of that one moment
is.
Learn to accept yourself
as you are.
Then begin your own rebuilding
by expanding your horizons.

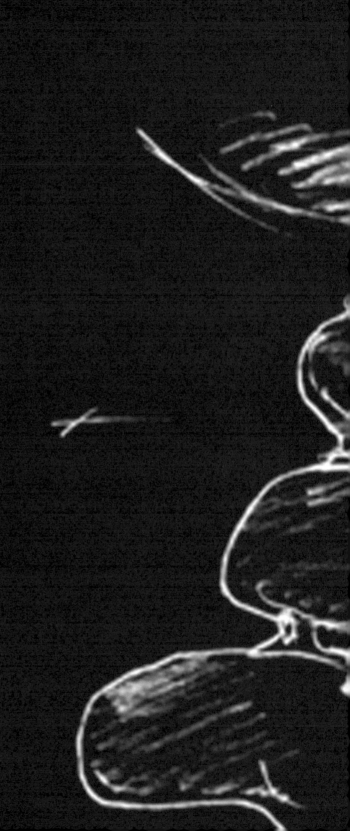

U nderstand your body. That is the sole purpose of this book. Do not attempt to treat yourself for any subluxation or lesion or allow anyone but a trained and board qualified doctor or chiropractor to treat you.

These pages and illustrations are a guide, a map to follow on your quest for health and happiness.

SLEEP

You exercise regularly. You even enjoy three meals a day. Yet, you are barely able to get through the day. What's the cause of this? Sleepless or restless nights probably have something to do with it.

You are getting less sleep because you choose to do more during the day. You have given up the hours your mind and body need to sleep, not just to rest. You may be a member of that group of people who would like to sleep more but just can't. Sleep is based on individual need. If you feel tired during the day, you likely need more sleep.

Too little sleep will drain your mental, emotional, and physical energy. Whenever a patient came to see me and I noticed they were "drained," I left them to sleep after a treatment at least 20-30 minutes. They did not realize that too little sleep was a source of deprivation during their business and social life.

As a woman, you likely experience difficulty in falling asleep, or once having fallen asleep, in staying asleep. If this occurs, you may need to consult your doctor as this may be the result of hormonal changes. You may notice this sleepless experience as more pronounced at the beginning of your menstrual cycle. The quality of sleep begins to lessen with age and by the time you reach age 60 sleeplessness becomes more common. The need for sleep does not decrease with age, but your ability to sleep changes. When your ability to sleep is disrupted for more than a month, you should seek medical attention.

. . . .

CAUSE OF SLEEPLESSNESS

Your ability to sleep may be the result of medical causes such as arthritis, breathing difficulties, back pain, irregular heart beat, drugs, alcohol, caffeine or other stimulants. Among the sleep-inhibiting drugs are beta-blockers, anti-depressants, decongestants, medications taken for asthma or cold, and thyroid hormone replacement medications. Also, do not discount the impact on sleep from depression, job-related changes, jet lag and your decision to limit sleep so that you can do more with your time in as burning the candle at both ends.

SOLUTIONS

Helpful sleep aids include: medications before bedtime, counting sheep, performing deep breathing exercises, a cup of milk (it contains trypotophan, a sleep-inducing amino acid), or eating a piece of fish, a banana, or a turkey patty before you go to sleep. Avoid soft drinks before sleep, as the caffeine included in these may last during the entire time you need to sleep. Avoid alcohol. Avoid naps during the day. If you must nap, do so early in the afternoon and for no more than 20-30 minutes.

The most important solution to sleep deprivation is the increase of exercise. It promotes good health and a full night's sleep. I always recommended walking to all my patients, a minimum of 20 minutes 3 times a week. Build up walking time by adding five minutes weekly. Walking should be done three to four hours before bedtime. Exercise wakes up your endorphins and increases your perceived need to quiet down.

Make sure your mattress is right for your back. A mattress that is too soft or too hard will cause neck pains and overall back pains, especially hip pains while you are on your side. If you sleep on your back all night, let your pillow be a firm or medium type. If you sleep on your side, use a firm pillow. And if you sleep on your stomach, use a soft pillow.

Learn habits just as you did when you were a child. You had a ritual, such as brushing your teeth. Someone may have read you a bedtime story. (You can read a book.) Take a lukewarm shower or a bath two hours before you go to bed. (Do not take a hot bath or shower as you will not be able to sleep. In addition, hot water dries out your skin. And, if you suffer from high blood pressure, heat is the worst thing for you.) Keep a regular routine. Don't read in bed or write checks. Use your bed for sleep and love. Keep your feet warm. Warmth induces sleep.

1. Develop good sleep habits
2. Avoid naps, if possible
3. Avoid alcohol late in the evening
4. Avoid caffeine late in the afternoon or evening
5 Never go to bed on an empty stomach or on an overstuffed one
6. If you smoke, don't smoke for at least 3 hours before bedtime
7. Establish a routine before bedtime
8. If you use an alarm clock, face it away from your eye
9. Check with your physician to see if your medication affects sleep
10. Keep your bedroom quiet
11. Maintain a regular schedule for sleep every day
12. Remember your bedroom is for sleep and love

G ETTING H ELP

If you are unable to resolve your sleep problem, consult your health care provider. Make sleep a #1 priority in the maintenance of health. You will benefit!

P OOR S LEEP AND N ERVOUS E XHAUSTION

Remedy

Oats

Eat oats daily as a hot cereal and before going to bed. Oats encourage a good night's sleep, especially for people suffering from nervous tension.

....

Hops

When the mind refuses to "switch off," hops is excellent. Hops relaxes the mind and is effective against insomnia.

OSTEOPOROSIS

Protect your bones. Your bones weaken with age or as a result of bad posture. You can prevent osteoporosis. If you already have the disease, remember there are treatments.

You know someone—or you are someone—an elderly man or woman with a stooped upper back, whose head is bent down as if looking for something on the ground. This person was taller, much taller, than at present. This condition occurs as old age sets in. In my practice I have found that this condition is not a necessity of aging. I have had patients in their 90s who have been helped and were able to regain their straight posture without difficulty. I was able to help them first structurally, then by teaching them how to maintain their new height and posture.

This stooped condition reveals an osteoporaic condition that is a sign of weak bones. These elderly persons' stooped posture has caused several small fractures in the spinal bones (vertebrae) which have become fragile due to thinning. These small fractures in the spine caused a decrease in height and rounding of the shoulders. What could happen to this elderly woman or man is a fall and consequently the break of the pelvic bone or one or both hips. This is actually a probability. More women have thinned-out spinal bones than men. Broken bones can and do cause disability and sometimes death.

The entire skeleton is as much alive as the liver or the heart. I have spoken before about the age of a person as determined by the age of the cells in the body. The cells of the skeleton must be kept healthy. These include those cells that make bones and those that dissolve bones.

The bones in your body are constantly undergoing renewal. Every bone is rejuvenated within the body several times during a person's lifetime. During childhood and teenage years most bone mass develops, but bones continue to grow in density (thickness) even after they stop growing in size. Most people reach their peak bone density between the ages of 20-25. After that, bone begins to break down faster than new bone is formed. For women, bone loss speeds up after menopause when the ovaries stop introducing estrogen, which protects against bone loss.

Women can lose up to a fifth of their bone mass in the seven years after menopause, thereby increasing their risk of osteoporosis. Men, too, are at risk of osteoporosis as they age. It is not natural to get osteoporosis even while it is natural to get older. Osteoporosis can also affect younger people. Young women with eating disorders or those who take certain kinds of medication that interfere with calcium absorption are at higher risk.

The thinning of bones or osteoporosis occurs without announcing its onset; it is a thief in the night. You may have osteoporosis without knowing about it until you fall and break a bone. If you are over 50 and a woman, you are more prone to bone breakage from osteoporosis than if you are a man of the same age.

Hip fractures can be disabling, requiring long-term care. Wrist fractures, as well, can be disabling making simple tasks difficult even in maintaining personal hygiene. One in three men are at risk of suffering a hip fracture from osteoporosis. Because you are a man, you have a larger skeleton, do not go through menopause, and so are less susceptible to osteoporosis.

Low levels of sex hormones in all men at any age place them at risk in a similar way as women to acquire osteoporosis; so do other chronic diseases that alter hormonal levels as well as long-term uses of certain medications.

WHO IS AT RISK?

In addition to advanced age, you are at risk for osteoporosis if you:

1. are female

2. are Asian or Caucasian (all women of all races have higher incidence of osteoporosis though)

3. are thin or have a small frame

4. eat poorly and have a low calcium intake

5. experienced menopause before age 45 or had your ovaries removed surgically

6. have a family history of the disease

7. live a sedentary lifestyle

8. have a low estrogen level

9. smoke

10. take certain medications that can interfere with calcium absorption when taken for a long time or at high doses

11. are a child who lives in a country where a nutritious diet is unavailable

Good news! Osteoporosis can be prevented. Diet and lifestyle changes can prevent bone loss.

FALLS

Preventing falls does not prevent osteoporosis but it does prevent broken hips and other fractures that cause disability at an age beyond 50 or in younger people with weak bones. Most falls occur at home.

Bathrooms: Install grab bars and nonskid tape in the tub or shower.

Floors: Remove throw rugs, get rid of cords that are in the way when you walk. Make sure carpets are secure.

Halls and stairways: Provide sufficient lighting. Put a night light in the bathroom. During the night, turn on a light before you take a step.

Kitchen: Clean all spills right away, whether water or oil. Use non-skid rubber mats near sink or stove, wear rubber soled shoes. Be cautious in consuming alcohol while working in your kitchen. Consult your physician regarding medication if you work in the kitchen; these may cause dizziness and cause a fall.

Osteoporosis begins to develop before you are old. It is preventable early in life, especially during childhood. Exercise and a calcium-rich diet early in childhood build healthy and strong bones. What should you do?

1. Eat a diet rich in calcium and Vitamin D.
2. Do exercise that supports your weight and use your arms when needed to support yourself.
3. Watch your lifestyle: do not do anything in excess.
4. Limit alcohol.
5. Don't smoke.
6. Check your bone density regularly by seeing your physician.
7. When necessary, take medication for bone-loss prevention and restoration.

Most important is diet. Almost all calcium in the body is in the bones and in your teeth. Your blood contains a small amount in order to regulate your heart beat and blood clot formation. If you fail to consume enough calcium, your body will take it from your bones to maintain blood levels. This will weaken your bones over a period of time.

The richest source of dietary calcium are dairy products, dark green leafy vegetables, grains, beans, peas, lentils, soy foods, oranges and orange juice.
Getting enough calcium depends on your body's ability to absorb calcium. Your body needs Vitamin D, which comes from sunlight and from food. Sunscreen blocks absorption of Vitamin D. Milk is fortified with Vitamin D. Eggs, margarine, fatty fish, and oleo also contain Vitamin D.

A high protein diet causes the body to lose more calcium in the urine. If you eat more protein, you will have less calcium. Sodium and caffeine increase calcium loss through urine. Take it easy with the salt and drink less coffee.

Use your muscles or you will lose them. Use your bones or you will lose them. The more you use your bones, the stronger they will get. Your legs must carry your weight. Therefore, walking is your #1 exercise. Climb stairs or dance. If you use a bicycle, or if you swim, these are not weight-bearing exercises. These are good for your heart, lungs and muscles.

Find an activity you enjoy. But walk and walk some more. All activity is beneficial for you. All inactivity is wrong for you and puts you at risk for osteoporosis. If you are a young woman, the only time exercise is bad for you is when exercise stops you from having a period. Then you have low estrogen and have experienced calcium loss. And, smoking produces lower levels of estrogen and less absorption of calcium.

You cannot cure osteoporosis, but medication can reduce bone loss, thereby reducing the risk of spinal and hip fractures. Consult your physician regarding medications. In the meantime, exercise and eat well and follow the suggestions made here.

EXERCISE

What does exercise mean to you? Does it mean simply placing an extra load on the human frame? That would be tension. Do you need more tension in your daily life? I should hope not. Your daily exercise should begin by being touched by and by you touching someone. All living beings want to be touched. Infants develop more positively when they are touched. Children desire to be hugged. As adults, this need should not be dismissed. Health is strengthened by touch. The human hand conveys the intent of the heart and the mind. Exercise to live and enjoy life, not just to punish the body.

When you wake up in the morning after a night of not sleeping well, or if you have an upset stomach, do not jump into push-ups to make yourself feel better. Touch someone, hug someone, even yourself. Your own body needs to be touched. Doing this is the first exercise of well being; it is essential to start the day right.

Before you get dressed in the morning, begin by touching your lumbar muscles. With your fingers, move your muscles up and down, and then press them together. This will relax you for the day. Then move the muscles of your buttocks with vigor. Your sciatic nerve pain runs through here to your leg. Move to the back of your head and massage your neck and head. Now you can get dressed. You have begun with a positive approach to the day.

FATIGUE

Get rid of that tired feeling by being active. Boredom causes stress. Get rid of it. Be happy each day; find something to do. Do something for someone else. Don't do it for money or personal gain. Do it for the sake of doing it. Feeling good needs practice, so does boredom. The more you practice being bored, the more you will feel useless to yourself and to others.

SHARE YOURSELF WITH SOMEONE

If one phase of your life is not pleasing to you, change it! A dull existence is not truly living. Do something about it. Share yourself. Get rid of your grudge. Grudges cause anger, hatred, envy, and resentment. These will all create fatigue. As long as you can breathe you can overcome boredom and fatigue.

YOUR EYES AND YOUR EARS

The eye of the mind is reason.

You should be aware that your eyes and ears determine how your body behaves. Always keep your eyes two degrees above the horizon. This will cause your body to straighten out. Your ears will then become more attuned to your surroundings. Your steps will become more sure as you walk toward the door to leave your house. By being more sure footed, you have turned on the machinery of good health. With this attitude, you create a feeling of confidence and assure yourself that the balance of the day will be productive. As you have begun to exercise your attitude, you will exercise the muscles of your mind and your emotions at the same time.

Your ears perform the same function as your eyes, especially in darkness. It is the ear by which you are learning to understand and master the world outside. You hear the words of love but you cannot see the words of love. Appreciate what you do have, and remember, the ear cannot defend itself, but your tongue can.

By keeping your eyes high and by tuning your ears to your surroundings, you have started using yourself. This is important: Self-conscious awareness is key for this day and every day, for the rest of your life.

··

WALKING

For decades I have taught my patients that the best exercise is what comes naturally. Walking is the most obvious exercise that comes naturally: It places no extra load on your body. Walking is safe.

A walking machine will strain your back somewhat whereas a walk in the park will not. A walking machine is a mechanical device which requires you to walk at the speed set on the machine. This is stressful to the human spine and sooner or later this stress will show. The ground does not set the pace for your walk outside. You set the pace. Therefore, the ground cannot hurt you but the machine can.

The purpose of walking is to accumulate an oxygen reserve in your body and increase your ability to endure the stresses of the day. In walking, you exercise the whole body, not just the muscles but your entire circulatory system as well.

Bicycling is next-best in terms of valuable exercise. A regular bike is best, although a stationary bicycle can be used to improve the cardiovascular system.

Any exercise that tears a joint or causes injury to the human body should be avoided. As I have stated before, the muscles should be able to support your own body weight. Tennis, volleyball, and racquetball are good cardiovascular workouts, but they will not develop the muscles needed to carry the weight of the body.

In conjunction with a healthy diet, exercise can help you maintain good health by lowering your cholesterol, controlling high blood pressure, and controlling the body's blood sugar levels. Remember, exercise should increase the oxygen reserve in your body and develop your muscles to support your own normal body weight.

The exercises I recommend throughout the book are a guide to help you. Try to invent exercises yourself that are a comfort to your body. Never punish your body by forcing it to perform a certain move or movements. The other purpose of exercise is to prevent shortening of the muscles. Slow stretching, such as the movements performed in Tai Chi, are beneficial. Violent exercise is a no-no!

I gave the following exercise to my patients to help them strengthen their backs. You can do this exercise in bed or on the floor; but do it exactly as outlined. Here, again, it is the oxygen reserve that is built up. The breath is the most important feature of the exercise.

Phase I:

1. Lie on your back with a pillow (optional) under the head.

2. Place your hands by your side in a relaxed manner.

3. Now take a deep breath. Let your stomach relax and bulge out by allowing your diaphragm to push the organs below it to drop down.

4. While holding your breath, count to 60. At first, you will not be able to hold your breath for very long. Don't worry; this will improve in time.

5. Exhale and relax. Do this exercise for one week before you attempt Phase II. Do this two times a day and build up to ten repetitions each time.

Phase II:

Do the same as Phase I; but as you inhale and hold your breath, dig your heels into your mattress and tighten the muscles of your limbs at the same time.

Note: Hold your breath as long as possible. You should be able to hold your breath at least one minute (two minutes after long practice). Do this for one week twice a day. Build up to ten times each time. You will notice that your stomach muscles and your thigh muscles will become firm. Remember, it is not the number of times you do the exercise, but how long you hold your breath that's important.

Phase III:

Now add the following:

1. Turn your head to the right. As you inhale, dig your ankles into the mattress, then elevate your shoulder three inches from the mattress. Keep your head to the right. When finished, exhale and relax.

2. Do the same on the left. Turn your head to the left and begin.

   Do not sit up with your head straight. You will tighten your spinal cord this way.

· ·

When your head is turned, you relax the spinal cord. You do not want to make a full sit up; lift yourself only three inches off the bed or floor. In one week your stomach muscles will be tight and strong. Build up to ten repetitions twice a day. Do these exercises for two months before you do Phase IV.

Do not attempt to do this exercise without progressively building up from Phases I, II, and III. If you skip immediately to Phase IV, you are bound to strain yourself. All beginnings are slow and safe. Good beginnings insure good progress.

Phase IV:

1. Lie on your stomach, with your head toward the foot of your bed. Your head should slightly clear the bed so that you can breathe freely.
2. Dig your toes into the mattress.
3. Keep your hands by your sides.
4. Inhale deeply as before.
5. Tighten your limbs as your toes press down on the mattress.
6. Exhale.

This is a safe back exercise to add to your walking.

SIMPLE RULES TO FOLLOW

A mother walked into my office one day seeking relief from a headache. She was a long-standing patient of mine. When I saw her, she looked downhearted, with bags under her eyes. She seemed demoralized.

"Nancy" (not her real name), I said, "What's wrong?"

"I haven't slept well for six months, since my baby was born," she answered. "She cries day and night. I have taken her to all kinds of doctors, and they can't figure out why. They tell me she's fine. But she can't be fine. I'm beginning to resent her. And, that's not right."

I interrupted her, and asked, "Was she by any chance a breech delivery?"

"Yes."

"Bring her in," I said. "I think I will be able to stop her crying."

Later that day, when she appeared with the child in my office, I saw that the child's head was tilted to one side. With one finger I was able to lift her tiny head back to its proper place, and the child stopped crying from pain.

The head is balanced on two small plates called "condyles." In cases of trauma or a wrong move, the head can move off one or both condyles, compressing the vertebral artery before it enters the foramen magnum (the opening to the skull). This pressure causes pain as the blood is forced into the brain. It is very important that you do not twist or turn you head or anyone's head, or allow an untrained or unlicensed person to touch you or any member of your family.

Breech delivery can cause problems in the neck and head, and, as a result of imbalance, affect the low back of an infant if it is not taken care of right away. To be aware is to be forewarned. Your neck is the support of the head. Take good care of it.

1. Do not stand on your neck.

2. Do not wrestle if you do not have to.

3. Do not carry heavy objects on your head.

4. Do not hang with your feet dangling and the rest of your body off the floor (e.g., from a bar at the gym). You may do hand stands but not head stands.

When a child falls off the bed, her head may become twisted on her neck, and problems can develop. Do not neglect that fall.

1. Check to see if the head is level on both sides.

2. Determine whether the child feels dizzy or sleepy.

3. Do not let the child go to sleep after a fall on the head or a twist of the neck. Keep the child awake for quite a while.

4. Phone your doctor and report the incident. Seek his/her advice.

I was awakened many times after midnight by patients when their children fell out of bed and twisted their neck or head. The parents were aware of the need to consult a professional for the sake of their children.

There are conditions during which trauma to the head and neck frequently occur, such as bicycling, horseback riding, motorcycle riding, climbing a fence or a tree.

Rule #1:

- When riding a bicycle, always wear a helmet.
- When horseback riding, always wear a helmet.
- When motorcycle riding, always wear a helmet.
- When climbing a tree or a fence, always wear a helmet.

Rule #2:

- When a fall occurs, always check yourself or check your children, not just for bruises, cuts, and superficial injuries, but also for possible tissue irritation, internal injuries, ligamentous strains, sprains, or concussions.

Rule #3:

- When a child falls too frequently, or when an adult falls frequently, check the eyes, each one separately. In children under three years, check to be sure that both eyes are being used equally. The child may look through one eye only, and not both at the same time. You can test your child's eyes yourself. Do not wait until the child says to you, "I hurt the eye I see through." Then it will be too late. Prevention is half the battle in preserving good health.

Rule #4:

- Always check the mobility of your arms, legs, hands and feet. In your children, make it a habit before they are tucked in for the night. Check the movements of their limbs as well. Make sure you ask them if they hurt anywhere. Also, ask if they feel good or sad, or if anything is bothering them. This will show them that you care and that you love them. Security and stability in their lives are some thing you must give them each day.

Rule #5:

- Do not take yourself or any member of your family or friends for granted. Show interest in them and in yourself. Your body is your only means of communicating with the world, outside and inside of your self.

Rule #6:

We as human beings:

- have the capacity for perpetual growth in every way—intellectually, emotionally, physically, and spiritually.
- need discipline in our daily life, not just in our work, but also in taking care of our bodies, our minds, and our feelings.
- . have the capacity to create harmony within ourselves, among the body, mind and emotions. The recognition of this harmony is necessary before we can be in harmony with any other human being or with the natural order of things around us.

Rule #7:

- As the actions of physical substances produce light in the physical world, so does your life produce the light of your consciousness with awareness that you are a human being. This awareness makes you responsible for yourself, for what you do to yourself and to others.

RELAX YOUR BODY WITHOUT EFFORT

I taught this exercise to my patients. You can do it at anytime, anywhere you have a straight back chair and a wall or its equivalent. When you finish this simple exercise, you will be refreshed and totally relaxed. Here is what you need to do:

1. Place your chair next to a wall.
   a. Make a fist with your left hand.

b. Place your fist, fingers downward, against the wall.

c. Pull, with your right hand, the back of the chair against your fist.

d. You should be able to move your fist freely between the wall and the back of the chair. (It shouldn't be wedged tightly against the wall.) Your fist is the anatomical measure for your neck's ability to bend backward without strain.

2. Sit on the chair as straight as possible.

   a. Place the soles of your feet together so that they face one another.

   b. Your ankles should now feel relaxed.

   c. Place your arms by your side and allow them to hang effortlessly.

3. Now bend your head back and let it rest on the wall.

   a. Close your eyes and sit quietly.

   b. Do not count or visualize anything.

   c. Sit as long as you enjoy it. Within two minutes, you will be relaxed completely.

Make sure that your head is one fist away from the wall. If you are not comfortable, check your chair against your fist, and adjust the distance of the chair from the wall. You can do this exercise as often as you want.

HOW TO SIT AND HOW TO GET UP

Very few people know how to sit down correctly and how to rise from a chair, sofa, or bench properly. Consequently, injury to the low back frequently occurs. I taught most of my patients how to sit and get up from a chair properly.

This is what you need to know:

1. When sitting down or getting up from a sitting position, place both hands on your thighs, keeping your head up.

2. Do not look down. The chair or sofa is behind you. Looking down tightens the spinal cord and causes tension throughout your body.

3. Press on your thighs and inhale at the same time.

4. Hold your breath and sit down.

5. Exhale and relax by placing the soles of your feet together. Do not keep the soles of your feet flat on the floor, or you will not be able to relax.

6. To get up, inhale and flatten your feet.

7. At the same time, place your hands on your knees, not on your thighs. Press down, keeping your head up. Hold your breath and proceed to stand up.

8. Exhale and proceed to stand or walk.

These simple rules will protect your back from injury. Remember to hold your breath whenever you make a move. Inhaling is the silent signal to your body that you are going to move. The body will reward you by protecting itself against your sudden decisions by not disabling you.

How to Get Out of Bed

The same rules apply in getting out of bed. Be careful!

1. Never sit up in bed with your head held straight, looking up or ahead.

2. Turn to the side where you get out of bed.

3. If you are getting out of bed on the left side, place your right hand opposite your left shoulder. If from the right, use the left hand.

4. Take a deep breath, pushing at the same time with your right hand. Now swing your legs out of bed and exhale.

5. Remember to pull your chin toward your chest before standing up. You will avoid getting dizzy this way. Hold your chin close to your chest and shorten the distance of your head from your heart. You will avoid falling and injuring yourself.

Remember, take a deep breath before making a move with your body.

Whenever you can say "Yes"
to life—
You have already said Yes
to All Life

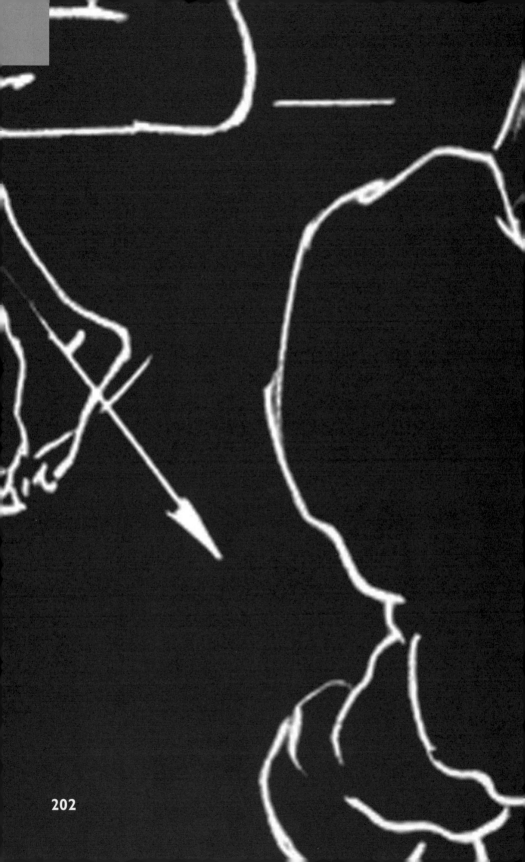

202

CONCLUSION

Truth is its own light
and
Understanding is the ointment
that
Brings healing and value
to
Heart and mind
that
Is in need
Remember!
Learning alone
is
not yet understanding

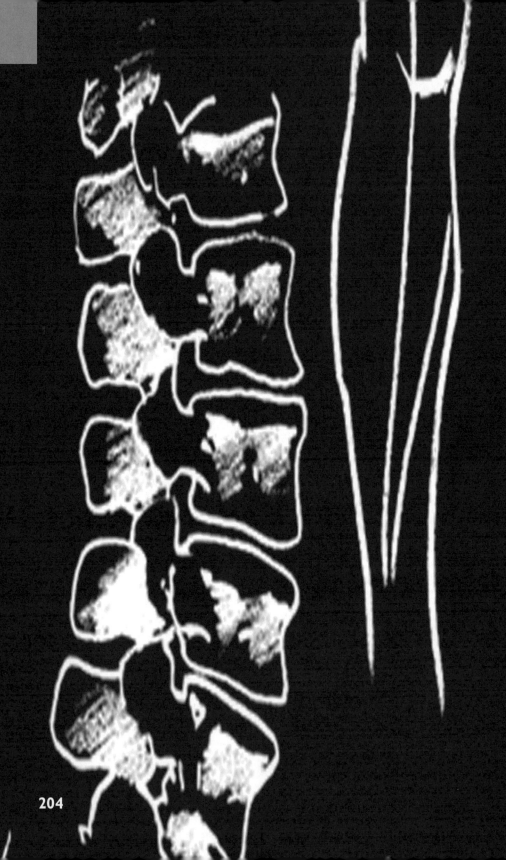

204

I have written this book as a guide to help you better understand your body and yourself. Your life must be allowed to have a say in your daily affairs. Your mind needs education and discipline. The life in you knows it all. It built you up in your mother's womb. We need to discover its wisdom.

I have learned over the years that man on this earth is the chief glory among the creations and manifestations of all life. No animal has been fashioned to desire a spiritual life. You and I as human beings, as human spirits, have the power to build the spiritual entity. An animal is like a vessel filled with water. No more can be put into them. ALL LIFE quickened them by his wisdom and his hand. As a drop of water has no power before the sun, so is the spirit of an animal before the light of His countenance. But to the human spirit He gave life everlasting in the desire for constant progress. He gave no progress to a stone, or to the tree, or to an animal, or to the waters of the ocean, regardless of how often they form clouds and fall back as rain and run to the rivers and back to the ocean, again and again.

The human spirit was brought into the world as a conscious person, and was nourished by ALL LIFE. Soon, man walked upright, and now he holds his head high, never to return to crawling on the belly or walking with the head bent to the ground.

Let the small spark of human wisdom and decency within your life grow into a great sun of light. Be strong. Never seek your own glory, for ease, or rest. Seek wisdom to be wise, to be just. Be quick to extend yourself to those in need. Do it without hesitation. Do not doubt the judgment of your life, and you will never again doubt your own. In the silence of your heart, keep on hoping, forever. And the star of faith will grow in you eternally, and the wisdom of ALL LIFE shall be your crown.

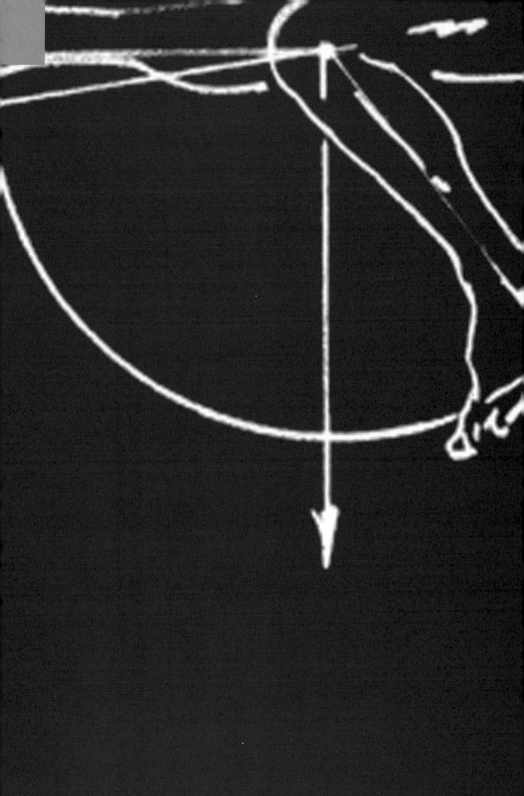

APPENDIX:

ANATOMICAL OVERVIEW

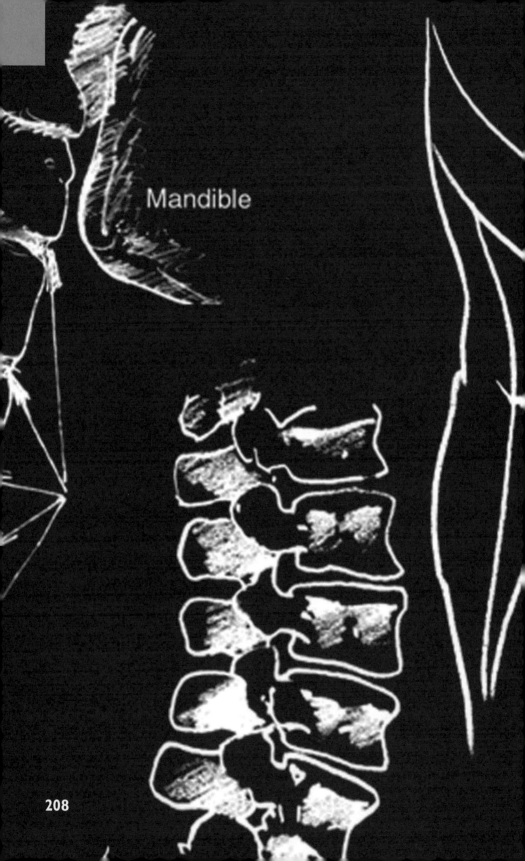

Mandible

J OINT   M OVEMENTS

Levers

J There are several varieties of movement:

    1. Adduction: Backward toward the spine.

    2. Abduction: Forward and away from the spine.

    3. Rotation upward: Turning the glenoid cavity upward and the scapula away from the spine. (The glenoid cavity is a socket into which the upper arm is attached to the shoulder blade.)

4   Rotation downward: Returning the scapula to the spine and the glenoid cavity to its normal position.

5   Elevation: Hunching the shoulders.

6   Depression: Returning to normal position.

The pivotal point of all movements is at the junction of your collarbone (clavicle) and your sternum (breast plate).

Hip Joint

Bones:

    The femur (the thigh) fits into the acetabulum (a cup-shaped cavity on the side of the hipbone) of the pelvic bones.

Movements:

    Flexion: The femur moves forward on the pelvis.

    Extension: The femur returns to position.

    Abduction: The femur moves to the side or lifting the leg sideward.

    Adduction: The femur returns to position.

    Rotation outward: The foot moves outward.

    Rotation inward: The foot returns to position.

Knee Joint

Bones:

Femur and tibia (the leg), with patella (kneecap) resting on front of the joint formed.

Movements:

Flexion or bending of a knee.

Extension or straightening the knee.

Observation:

The knee is a hinge joint.

Muscles affecting the hip and knee:

Rectus femoris knee extensor

Sartorius knee flexor

Biceps femoris knee flexor

Semitendinous knee flexor

Semimembranous knee flexor

Gracilis knee flexor

Ankle Joint

Bones:

Tibia, fibula, and astragalus (ankle)

Movements:

Elevation: The top of the foot moves toward the shinbone.

Depression: The sole of the foot moves downward.

Pronation: The sole turns outward.

Supination: The sole turn inward.

Observation: The tibia moves on the astragalus. The body weight is transferred from the tibia to the astragalus to the calcaneum (heel bone), the weight-bearing bones.

The Foot

Movements:

Metatarsals on tarsals and phalanges on metatarsals.

Lateral flexion: Drawing the toes and front part of the foot toward the calcaneum.

Extension: Return.

Observation:

The importance of these movements cannot be overemphasized. The bones and ligaments alone cannot maintain arch structure and movement. The muscles producing these movements are important in the maintenance of the arches. The toes used effectively give balance, poise, and strength to the arches.

The Trunk

Bones:

Vertebrae are superimposed on each other. The pelvis is involved in movements of the vertebrae because of the close connection between the ilium (pelvis) and the sacrum (lower back) at the lower spinal column. As the pelvis teeters forward or backward on the femur, it determines the degree of lumbar curve.

Movements:

Flexion of the trunk: Movement of the xiphoid cartilage (a small piece of cartilage on the end of your chest plate) toward the pubis or the pubis toward the xiphoid.

Extension:

Return or separation of the xiphoid and the pubis

Lateral flexion (left or right): Movement of your shoulder toward either hip.

Rotation of the trunk: Turning of the vertebrae on each other on a horizontal plane.

Observation:

The movement of vertebrae on each other in any direction is limited. The great range of movement in your trunk is carried out by the head on the spine and your pelvis on the femur.

Seek a personal relationship
with ALL LIFE
and in turn with the individual
human being and humanity at large.
This way your whole being
is renewed each moment
YOU Live.

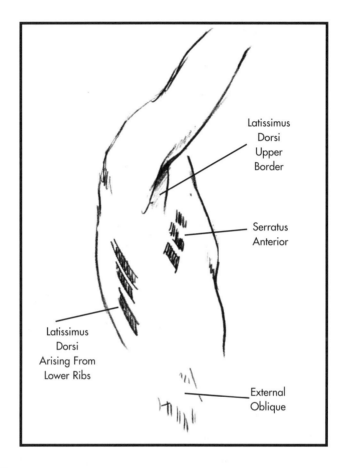

Latissimus Dorsi Upper Border

Serratus Anterior

Latissimus Dorsi Arising From Lower Ribs

External Oblique

MUSCLE

You move. You jump. You walk. You dance. You hug. You hold hands. You kiss. You cry. You touch. You feel. You smile. You sit. You stand. You look. You hear. What performs these actions?

Where does the power come from? Your life, of course. But what does your life use to give you the power to move? Muscle tissue!

Muscle tissue endows you with the power of movement. You have three types of muscles in your body: involuntary, cardiac, and voluntary.

Plain, or involuntary, muscle is found in the walls of your viscera, all vessels and glands, in the iris and ciliary muscles (a muscle of the eye); if you are a male, in the dartos (contractible tissue under the skin of the scrotum) and in the arrectores pilorum in your penis. Your cardiac or heart muscle varies in the speed of its contraction. For example, the heart of a canary beats 1000 times to the elephant's 250 beats per minute. If you are an athlete, your heart at rest may be 45 beats per minute, 80 with moderate effort, and 180 with maximum effort.

Your voluntary or skeletal muscle makes up 40% of your body weight and consists of fibers. By exercising, you increase the thickness of the existing muscle fibers, but the number of fibers remains constant. When extensive injury occurs for any reason, it results in a fibrous tissue substitute. These may be repaired by regeneration from the intact ends. All the vessels in your body are accompanied by nerves that enter the muscles usually at a definite line or slight cleft, called the neurovascular hilum (a pit giving entrance or exit to vessels or nerves). Your muscles, however, also receive numerous vessels at other points almost constantly.

NEUROMOTOR UNIT

Joints move like levers. Gravity pressure on the body begins at the ankles, knees, and by the second or third segment of the sacrum, in the area of lumbar #1, where the neck and the thoracic meet at cervical #7, and at the atlas where the head rests on the neck. When lifting, you must lift on the first lever. Balance on your toes, shifting your weight to your heels which carry most of the body weight; then on the knee, pushing upward; then on the hip. In this way, the back is never bent, but remains in the normal position. When lifting is done by bending forward, the weight will be between the thoracic (rib cage) #11 to L#1, the weakest part of the back. This is what leads to back pain.

In the application of levers to your body, the power is where the muscle attaches to the bone. A muscle has a place where it begins and where it ends. Where it begins is called "origin," where it ends is called "insertion", into a ligament or a tendon. In between these two points is the "belly" of the muscle. For example, in the elbow and in the ankle, the power is behind the joint.

C O M M O N   L E V E R S   I N   T H E   B O D Y

The biceps apply force between the fulcrum (the elbow joint) and the weight (the forearm).

A   S Y N O P S I S   O F   B O D Y   J O I N T S

A body joint is the junction between two or more bones admitting motion of one or more bones, allowing the motion of one or more of those bones. It is also the site of most athletic injuries, at the knee, ankle, and elbow joints.

Shoulder Girdle

Bones:

The clavicle (collarbone) and scapula (shoulder blade) move as a unit.

It is important very for you to understand how critical it is to protect your spine. Nerves to your muscles contain both motor and sensory fibers. Almost half are sensory. Bundles of these fibers divide until each motor nerve fiber supplies a definite group of muscle fiber. The number of muscle cells may be only five in a small muscle—for example, the muscle that provides the movement of your eyeball—compared to the 200 in the gluteus maximus muscle. Muscles, to be effective, work in relays or shifts. The motor unit system provides continuous activity without fatigue during light effort. The more vigorous the action, the more units are harnessed at the same time until, for maximal effort, all are activated.

Even at rest your muscles are under slight tension due in part to the activity of the motor unit system. Your sensory nerve fibers, by which you touch or taste, are nerve paths to the central nervous system for stimuli initiating the reflex controlling and coordinating muscular activity. All motor nerves excite the muscle to contraction.

ANATOMICAL OVERVIEW

NOMENCLATURE

All your muscles are named from their shape, size, structure, situation, directions, action, and attachment; for example, the biceps which flex your elbow, move food to your mouth; pectorals help in push-ups, regulating your shoulder blades' movements; and the sternomastoid, flexes the neck to move your head.

The attachment of a muscle at the origin is the more stable or fixed point, while the insertion is more mobile; but the roles may be reversed in different actions. In the muscles from the legs to the foot the insertions are usually fixed points.

Tendons act as buffers, protecting against the sudden strains and excessive speed in a limb. The elasticity of a tendon increases muscular action, such as in jumping.

Muscle tension. A muscle fiber, fully stretched or relaxed, may contract to almost half its length. The amount of shortening that a muscle may undergo depends upon the arrangement of fibers.

MUSCLES AND GRAVITY

Your muscles maintain your balance in the erect posture (against gravity). These are controlled by the central nervous system through reflexes in the spinal cord, from impulses arising from the muscles in your eyes, your skin, and your ears. Your posture depends upon attitude, by thinking straight. The line of the center of gravity in your body passes in front of your ankle joint, when your erect position is maintained by the activity of your calf muscles. At your hip and knee joints, your ligaments may take the strain against gravity before the muscles take over.

POWER, RANGE, AND SPEED

Your physical power depends on muscle fibers: The greater the number of fibers, the greater is their strength; the longer the fibers, the greater the range of your movement.

Speed, which varies with individual muscles, is a part of the intrinsic quality of the muscle itself. This is dependent on its biochemical and physiochemical constitution, and is not dependent entirely on the nervous system. For example, the smaller the ani-

216

mal, like a rabbit or squirrel, the more rapid the speed of its muscles. Again, the muscles that move your eyeball contract more rapidly than the muscles of your buttocks that move your thigh.

As in everything else in life, there is always a compromise made between the energy expended and the speed involved, depending on what function is required to be performed by the muscle. The blinking of your eyelid needs speed but little power, while your legs need more power.

Power, range, and speed of movements produced by a muscle depend on the number and length of the fibers. It is important to understand that when you perform isometric exercises, the tension of the muscles increase but the length remains the same.

Don't be a hero by trying to prove to yourself that you can lift something that weighs more than you can comfortably lift, as you cannot lift anything beyond your muscle strength!

VOLUNTARY MOVEMENT

The term "voluntary muscle" describes the nature of the movement of the executive or primary muscles. Your will orders a movement, but it cannot select the muscle required to perform that movement. A muscle, like a good soldier, never acts alone; it is assisted by companion muscles or other structures. Because of this association, those assisting or controlling the movements are known as the prime movers, antagonists, fixation muscles, and synergists.

Prime movers are the principal muscles actively producing a movement. Your biceps and brachialis of your upper arm are the prime movers in flexing your elbow.

Antagonists are in opposition to the prime movers, and are able to prevent or reverse a movement. They arrest, relaxing the prime mover as it contracts.

Relaxation is an important feature in all exercises. For example, when you touch your toes and your knees are straight, your hamstrings need to be relaxed. Exercise should be balanced to secure both the full contraction and the full relaxation of the muscle.

217

The more vigorous the action of the prime movers, the greater the resistance, and the more relaxed are the antagonists.

Fixation muscles steady one part, providing a firm base for movement by other muscles. For example, the muscles attached to your shoulder blade steady the bone so that the upper arm (humerus) may be moved upon the glenoid cavity.

Synergists (syn = together, ergein = to work) control movement at proximal (near) joints so that prime movers may exert their action upon a distal (far) joint. Your wrist, if it is extended, will enable your fingers to exercise a powerful grip.

FATIGUE

Do not abuse your body by too rigorous exercise. Muscular fatigue occurs with strenuous exercise because circulation is impeded. The site of fatigue is the muscle itself, not your central nervous system. When circulation is occluded, movement is difficult, as in a sudden heart attack during rigorous exercise.

In concluding this section on the muscular system, I must stress the importance to the reader, especially to physical trainers and physicians, that muscles reveal not just their nerve supply but also the condition of the nervous system. Keep adequate blood supply to the muscles and nerves. Without oxygen no nourishment can reach any of the organs and the body is a whole system of organs.

LIGAMENTS

Ligaments are composed mainly of bundles of collagenous fibers. They are white, shiny and silvery in appearance. They are flexible and pliant. They are tough, not yielding easily to force. They allow freedom of movement. In lower animals ligaments substitute for muscular power mainly in their neck. Moveable joints are covered by an articular capsule (a joint enclosed with a sac-like envelope). Muscles sometime act as ligaments, restraining certain movements of one joint. As an example: The shortness of the hamstring muscles prevents complete flexion of the hip unless the knee joint is also flexed so as to bring their attachments nearer together.

CERVICAL NERVES

You have seven cervical vertebrae but eight cervical nerves. Each of seven nerves passes above its corresponding vertebra; the eighth cervical nerve passes below the seventh cervical and above the first thoracic vertebrae. The first thoracic nerve runs beneath the first thoracic vertebrae so that there are twelve thoracic nerves into the five lumbar, five sacral, and one coccygeal. The vertebral name and number given to a pair of spinal nerves is also applied to the segment of the cord from which these nerves originate. The nerves supplying your arms and legs are large, but the upper sacral nerve is the largest in your body.

It is important to understand the function of the peripheral (outward) nerves.

The terminal branches divide into vascular, articular, muscular, and cutaneus twigs. The vascular twigs are efferent (motor) fibers which relieve arterial spasm. The articular twigs are somatic afferent proprioceptive in function which means that they supply your joints and ligaments.

The muscular branches carry somatic efferent (motor) fibers to your voluntary muscles but almost half of the fibers in these branches are proprioceptive (sending information concerning movement of the body). They also innervate your bones, especially the periosteum, a connective tissue covering the bones. These have bone-forming potential.

The cutaneous branches carry somatic afferent exteroceptive sensations (external stimuli receptors) in the skin reacting to touch, pressure, pain, heat, or cold. They also carry (autonomic) visceral fibers innervating the smooth muscle, glands and small blood vessels in the skin. When there is an injury to the autonomic fibers it can cause a decrease in sweating and an increased electrical resistance of the skin. Skin trophic (nutritive) changes take place with peripheral nerve injury, so the skin becomes smooth and pink. The capillary bed (minute vessels resembling hair) shines through the skin (which is thin) and the nails are also changed.

You should always ask yourself: What will happen if this nerve is injured due to my own negligence during daily activity or a wrong decision I make?

The phrenic nerve in your neck is the main motor nerve to your diaphragm. It is formed mainly by a branch from the fourth cervical nerve with additional branches from the third and fifth. Injury to this nerve results in paralysis of the diaphragm on the same side.

Peritonitis, or inflammation of the gall bladder, may irritate the phrenic endings in the central part of the diaphragmatic peritoneum (muscle membrane separating the abdominal and thoracic cavities and the membrane lining the abdominal and pelvic cavity) and pain may be experienced in the shoulder due to the root origins shared in common by the phrenic and subclavicular nerves. Watch those whiplash injuries to your neck—you may not feel the pain right away, but it will show up later.

You, a human being in the likeness
of ALL LIFE
capable of being a partner
in an inner dialogue
a person to whom ALL LIFE
can talk and one
who could answer Him!
YOU!
To whom He gave a spark
of Himself
and liberty to choose the path
you wish to travel on.
To His questions to your heart
patiently He awaits
a reply.

GLOSSARY

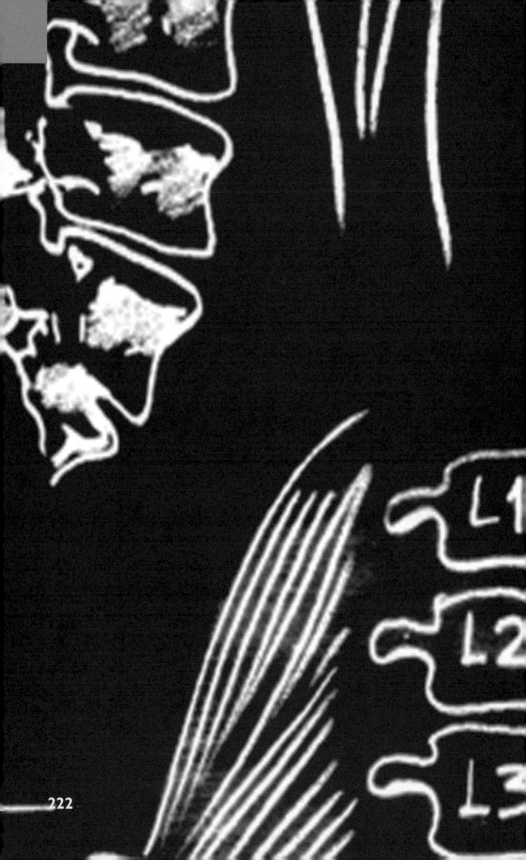

L1

L2

L3

Abduct	To draw away from the median plane.
Acetabulum	Cup-shaped cavity on the side of the hip bone.
Acute	Sharp, severe symptom of short duration.
Adduct	To draw toward the median plane.
Adjustment	To put in proper state or position.
Angina Pectoris	A pain caused by restricted blood supply due to hardening and narrowing of the coronary arteries supplying the heart muscle.
Aorta	The main trunk artery that receives blood from the left ventricle of the heart.
Aortic valve	The valve at the junction of the aorta or large artery and the left ventricle of the heart. It allows the blood to flow from the heart into the aorta and prevents back flow.
Arteriosclerosis	A disease in which the inner layer of the artery wall is made thick and irregular by deposits of fatty substances.
Arthritis	Inflammation of a joint.
Articulation	A joint.
Astragalus	Refers to the ankle.
Atrium	One of the two upper chambers of the heart. The right receives non-oxygenated blood from the body. The left receives oxygenated blood from the lungs.
Basilar	Base.
Biceps	A muscle having two heads.
Calcaneum	In the foot; the heel bone.
Capsule	An enclosing structure.
Cholesterol	A fat-like substance found in animal tissue. The normal level for men and women is assumed to be between 180 and 230 milligrams. Higher levels are considered as risk of coronary arteriosclerosis.
Compensation	Counterbalancing defects in structure or function.

Diabetes	A metabolic disorder in which the ability to use (oxidize) carbohydrates is more or less lost due to faulty pancreatic activity. Interferes with normal production of insulin.
Diaphragm	Any separating membrane or structure.
Eversion	A turning inside out; turning out the foot.
Fascia	A sheet or a band of fibrous tissue around a muscle and various body organs.
Femur	The thigh.
Glenoid	Resembling a pit or socket.
Gravity	Atmospheric pressure.
Hallux	The big toe.
Ilium	The pelvis.
Infra	Beneath.
Intervertebral disc	Between contiguous vertebrae.
Joint	The site or junction or union between two or more bones. One that admits motion.
Lesion	Pathological or traumatic discontinuity of tissue or loss of function of a part.
Ligaments	Fibrous tissue which supports and strengthens joints.
Meniscus	Somewhat crescent-shaped, such as the fibrocartilage in the knee joint.
Meta	Change; exchange; next.
Metatarsalgia	Pain in the metatarsus, the five miniature bones of the foot.
Mitral valve	A valve of two cusps located between the upper and lower chambers in the left side of the heart.
Myocardium	The muscular wall of the heart. The thickest of the three layers of the heart wall. It lies between the inner, larger (endocardium) and the outer layer (epicardium).
Myofibrositis	Replacement of muscle tissue by fibrous tissue.

224

Perecardium	A closed sac surrounding the heart and roots of the great vessels. The space inside the sac (the pericardial cavity), between the two walls, contains fluid that provides for smooth movements of the heart as it beats.
Peritoneum	Membrane lining the wall of the abdominal and pelvic cavities.
Pronograde	Walking with the body horizontal or near-horizontal, like an animal.
Psoitis	Inflammation of a psoas muscle or its sheet.
Pulmonary artery	The large artery that conveys non-oxygenated (venous) blood from the lower right chamber of the heart to the lungs.
Pulmonary valve	A valve formed by three cup-shaped membranes at the junction of the pulmonary artery and the right lower chamber of the heart (right ventricle).
Quadriceps	A muscle having four heads.
Reflex	A reflected movement or action (autonomic) mediated by the nervous system.
Sacrum	Lower back.
Semi	Half.
Septum	A dividing wall. A muscular wall dividing the left and right chambers of the heart.
Stenosis	A narrowing or stricture of an opening.
Sub	Under, near, almost, moderately.
Supra	Above, over.
Tarso	Edge.
Tarsus	The seven bones: talus, calcaneous, navicular, medial, intermediate, lateral cuniform, and cuboid, comprising the articulation between the foot and leg, the ankle or instep. Also refers to the cartilagenous plate forming the framework of either the upper or lower eyelid.

Teres	Long or round.
Thoracic	Pertains to the chest (thorax).
Tibia	The thigh.
Tricuspid valve	A valve consisting of three cusps or triangular segments located between the upper and lower chambers in the right side of the heart.
Ventricle	One of the main pumping chambers of the heart. The left ventricle pumps oxygenated blood through the arteries to the body. The right ventricle pumps non-oxygenated blood through the pulmonary artery to the lungs.